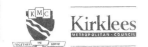

FEMALE CANCERS

BY THE SAME AUTHOR

Well Woman series

Female Cancers

A Complementary Approach

Jan de Vries

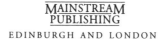

MAINSTREAM
PUBLISHING
EDINBURGH AND LONDON

First published in Great Britain in 2004 by
MAINSTREAM PUBLISHING COMPANY (EDINBURGH) LTD
7 Albany Street
Edinburgh EH1 3UG

ISBN 1 84018 847 2

A catalogue record for this book
is available from the British Library

Typeset in Garamond

Printed and bound in Great Britain by
Cox & Wyman Ltd

Contents

Chapter One

What is Cancer?

I was asked this question just a few days ago and it made me think that I should embark on writing a book dealing specifically with the cancers that affect women: breast cancer, ovarian cancer, cervical cancer and uterine cancer. I will also be discussing cancer in general, explaining what it is and how it may be treated and prevented. One of my previous books, *Cancer and Leukaemia*, also gives in-depth details of the various alternative or complementary ways in which cancer can be treated.

The question 'What is cancer?' came from a very healthy-looking lady who was approaching 50. Although she looked well, while she was speaking to me I could see that she had broken into a sweat and she told me that she was scared of getting cancer. I replied that fear is our worst enemy and as our mind is so much more powerful than our body, if we strongly focus it on something negative, there is a danger that we may cause whatever we are most dreading to happen. I will elaborate on this in Chapter Eight, on 'Cancer and the Mind'.

When the lady told me her story, it interested me and made me smile. She had been travelling on the underground when she had broken into a sweat: she was having a hot flush, a common and uncomfortable symptom of the menopause. A fellow lady passenger sitting across from her looked at her sympathetically. It is very sad in today's society that we cannot talk to one another any more, especially on the underground, as this is considered to be dangerous. Unless we know each other, we tend to refrain from becoming involved as certain situations can turn very nasty, as I once witnessed while travelling on the underground.

This lady noticed that the sympathetic woman opposite her had started to write a little note. As she stood to disembark, she handed this note over to her. It said, 'I can see your problem. I had a similar problem. HRT did not help and I also felt it was dangerous. May I advise you to see Jan de Vries for a consultation. A friend of mine advised me to see him. I am completely free of the perspiration problem now and my fear of cancer has gone.'

Many questions were raised regarding HRT and its possible relation to breast cancer when I took part in programmes with Gloria Hunniford on Radio 2 in the 1980s. In the 12 years that I appeared on these programmes, I reiterated my advice that if one can treat menopausal symptoms without HRT, one should do so. There are plenty of natural remedies which are just as effective. If you can be treated naturally, why would you want to take an artificial remedy?

In saying that, I would be lying if I claimed I had never advised a patient to take HRT. In some cases where there is absolutely no alternative, I recommend its use but I always inform patients that in the time I have been in practice, over 45 years, I have seen the side effects of HRT, including phlebitis, thrombosis and breast cancer. Even today, when a lot more has been learned by scientists about the hormone system, there is still not an endocrinologist or immunologist who knows exactly how the hormone system works. For this reason, it is important to take the more natural approach if at all possible.

Although the body's hormonal system is extremely complex and I will be discussing it throughout this book, I would like to digress for a short time to describe it in simple terms. It consists of a number of glands scattered around the body. Each gland is responsible for producing and secreting one or more specific chemicals which we call hormones. The hormonal system has a wide range of functions. It is involved with:

- Growth and development

- Regulation of mood
- Tissue function
- Sexual function and reproduction
- Use and storage of energy
- Maintenance of fluids, salt and sugars in the blood

Some examples of hormones are as follows:

HORMONE	SECRETED BY
Growth hormone	Pituitary
Thyroxine	Thyroid
Adrenaline, noradrenaline	Adrenals
Insulin	Pancreas
Testosterone	Testes
Oestrogen	Ovaries
Progesterone	Ovaries

Hormones are secreted into the bloodstream and, as a result, their effects are often seen far from the organ responsible for their production. The body's cells have receptors that attract specific hormones. This ensures that hormones work on the correct cell or organ. When the hormone is delivered to a cell, chemical messages are passed to the inside of that cell.

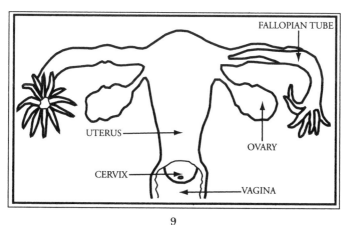

FALLOPIAN TUBE

UTERUS

OVARY

CERVIX

VAGINA

HOW THE FEMALE REPRODUCTIVE SYSTEM WORKS

The female reproductive system consists of a number of organs.

The ovaries are two walnut-sized structures that sit on either side of the uterus. Ovaries contain follicles in which eggs mature. Ovaries also produce hormones. When born, baby girls have about two million eggs in their ovaries.

The fallopian tubes are simple structures connecting the ovaries to the uterus. They allow eggs to be transported from the ovary to the uterus. Each fallopian tube is about 4 cm long.

The uterus, or womb, is a hollow muscular structure about the size of a pear. It is in the uterus that a fertilised egg implants and matures during pregnancy.

The cervix is the opening to the uterus through which the male sperm travels to fertilise an egg. It is through the cervix that the baby leaves the uterus.

The vagina is the passageway connecting the uterus to the outside world.

THE FEMALE REPRODUCTIVE HORMONES

Females have two specific hormones, known as oestrogen and progesterone, which help to run the reproductive system. These hormones are produced in the ovaries and secreted into the bloodstream. The production and secretion of the female reproductive hormones are controlled in turn by other hormones secreted by the pituitary gland, situated under the brain. These are known as follicle-stimulating hormone (FSH) and luteinising hormone (LH).

THE MENSTRUAL CYCLE

We commonly refer to menstruation as a 'period'. During menstruation, blood is lost from the uterus via the vagina. Menstruation lasts between three and seven days and occurs approximately every twenty-eight days. These are just average timescales; everyone is different. It is important that women get to know what is normal for them. Menstruation usually begins between the ages of ten and fourteen, although it can begin as late as eighteen. The first time a girl menstruates, it is known as the menarche. Menstruation usually stops when women are between 45 and 55 years old; this is known as the menopause. Altogether, most women menstruate about 550 times. Some women may experience a variety of symptoms around and after the menopause. These are commonly referred to as menopausal symptoms.

The whole menstrual cycle is very complicated. In essence, the following events happen during each cycle:

> FSH stimulates the production of oestrogen and growth of follicles which contain eggs.
>
> Oestrogen thickens the lining of the womb and rising oestrogen levels trigger the production of LH, which initiates an egg being released from one of the follicles in the ovary – this is known as ovulation.
>
> The egg matures and travels down the fallopian tube to the uterus.
>
> The ruptured follicle produces progesterone, which maintains the thickened womb lining.
>
> If a sperm fertilises the egg the woman becomes pregnant.
>
> If the egg is not fertilised, hormone levels fall and the unfertilised egg is passed out of the uterus. This is menstruation – when the lining of the uterus and the non-fertilised egg are released from the body.

Oestrogen is responsible for ovulation, while progesterone prepares the uterus for a fertilised egg.

You will hear people using the word 'premenstrual'. This is the term used to describe the few days before menstruation. During this time some women report a variety of physical and emotional symptoms. 'Postmenstrual' is not such a commonly used term. It is used to describe the days after menstruation, before ovulation begins again.

Levels of the female hormones change frequently in the body. This brings about the complicated processes that govern the female reproductive system.

It is to be noted that during some parts of the menstrual cycle, oestrogen levels are higher than progesterone. The reverse is true during other parts of the cycle. The healthy functioning of the whole menstrual cycle is dependent upon the correct balance of hormones at every single stage. It is the imbalance of these hormones that gives rise to difficulties.

WHAT GOES WRONG

In a normal, healthy menstrual cycle, oestrogen and progesterone levels rise and fall in a balanced way, depending upon the stage of the cycle. This balance is also important during the menopause, when both hormones show a natural decline.

The most common problems relating to the female hormonal system may be grouped as follows.

High Oestrogen

Generally, teenagers and young women with menstrual problems have oestrogen levels which are high relative to their progesterone levels. Symptoms experienced include heavy, painful periods, tender breasts, fluid retention, high anxiety, mood swings and nervous tension. In the longer term, high oestrogen levels may be a factor in the development of fibroids and endometriosis. Problems before and during menstruation are often referred to as PMT or PMS (Pre-Menstrual Tension or Pre-Menstrual Syndrome). The features of PMS are variable and different women experience them in different ways.

Low Oestrogen

Some women experience irregular periods, a lengthening of their cycles, low spirits or depression, weepiness and constipation before menstruation. Periods are often painless. These women are usually older, often approaching the menopause. However, with the widespread use of the mini-pill or progesterone-based hormone injections as contraception, younger women may also experience symptoms of low oestrogen.

Menopausal Problems

The menopause is not an illness – it is a natural phase of life that is necessary, unless you wish to continue having children in your 80s. During the menopause, levels of oestrogen and progesterone should fall gradually until your menstrual cycle ceases. If this fall is balanced, the menopause should be a relatively trouble-free time. However, if hormonal levels fall rapidly, or if one hormone falls more than another, unwanted symptoms will arise.

FACTORS THAT AFFECT THE SMOOTH RUNNING OF THE MENSTRUAL CYCLE

● A poor diet containing large quantities of sugar and caffeine will cause blood sugar levels to rise and fall dramatically, contributing to mood swings, cravings, fatigue and nervous irritation. A poor diet will also deprive you of nutrients that you need for a smooth cycle, e.g. zinc for mental balance, magnesium for relaxed muscles, vitamin B for reduced stress and chromium for keeping sugar cravings under control.

● Alcohol and nicotine consume vast quantities of useful nutrients such as those mentioned above.

● Stress uses up vitamin B and magnesium, making you more prone to irritation, anger and cramping pains. The adrenal glands produce inflammatory hormones in response to stress, making symptoms worse. Stress also weakens the adrenal glands, which has an adverse effect on the production of sex hormones.

● The liver is responsible for degrading oestrogen. If it is not working well, oestrogen levels will rise.

Let us return now to the menopause and HRT. I have advised hundreds of the people who come to see me to try natural methods. There is so much that can be done for hormonal imbalances, such as dietary management, exercise, natural medicine and natural hormone treatments. These are often very successful and I have seen good results in many patients who have tried such methods.

In the course of the lectures I have given over the years in 40 different states of the United States, I have been given feedback during the question and answer sessions that many ladies take HRT not only for help with symptoms such as perspiration, but to keep them looking young. They are afraid of getting wrinkles or crow's feet and believe HRT is the answer. In addition, they feel it will make them more attractive to the opposite sex. Nothing is further from the truth. Many problems have arisen because of such misconceptions. It always amazes me that it has taken so many years for the medical establishment to come to the conclusion that HRT has side effects. Even though the press might have exaggerated these side effects, there is definite evidence that problems have occurred with the use of HRT. This has come to the fore through recent research.

Let us revert to the question, 'What is cancer?' Basically, cancer is a condition in which cells are out of control. I often remind patients that cancer is like warfare. It can be compared to two opposing armies: the army of degenerative cells at war with the army of regenerative cells. If the former appears to be stronger, we have to provide the right materials and weapons for the army of regenerative cells to prop up their defences. A victory of the regenerative cells is then certainly not impossible. There is a wide range of natural weapons we can use to strengthen the army of regenerative cells and in this book I will outline some of these.

This is where complementary healthcare comes into its own: not only dietary management but also exercise and natural medicines, which I will talk about later in this book. A positive mind is also essential. Methods like Chinese breathing exercises, 'mind over matter' techniques and visualisation are all very important in the fight against cancer.

Cancer occurs when the cells, the 'building blocks' of the body, become diseased. Although these cells are different in each part of the body, they all either repair or reproduce themselves. There is therefore a lot one can do to control cancer by helping the regenerative cells. Normal cells look like an even plateau of little eggs with points in them – this is when tumours are benign. A tumour, however, when malignant, will grow out of this normal plateau like a muscle. In a benign tumour, the cells do not spread to other parts of the body, so we can then say they are not cancers. If they grow normally, there is no problem unless the tumour presses on surrounding organs. A malignant tumour has the ability to spread away from the original site. If the tumour is left untreated, it can invade and destroy surrounding tissues, or break away into a primary cancer condition and spread to other organs, such as the lymphatic system. When these cells reach yet another site, a new tumour can establish itself. It is always important to realise that cancer is a metabolic disease and that although there are more than 200 different types of cancer, each one has its own form and name, and each requires a specific treatment. Later in this book, I will go into more detail about the different cancers that can affect women. Now let us talk a little bit more about what cancer is.

How often have we witnessed the terror the very sound of the word 'cancer' strikes in today's society? Cancer does not respect status and will attack rich and poor, old and young. I was still very young when I first became aware of this dreaded disease. My younger sister was born during the winter of 1944–5 which in the Netherlands, where I originate from, is commonly referred to as the 'Hunger Winter', for obvious reasons. How well I remember that wintry, grim morning, with death and destruction all around us. My mother – a very brave woman – was conducting a meeting which was interrupted by sirens warning us of an air raid and when the all-clear sounded, she asked one of her friends to take me home with her, as she had gone into labour. The local doctor was informed and also the midwife.

Although still very small, I realised that something unusual was going on when I was taken away by my mother's friend. The subsequent birth of my little sister seemed like a ray of sunshine and hope in a world full of misery and danger. It was something that cheered us all up and to the adults it acted temporarily as a diversion from their worries about the war.

A day later I was back home again, once arrangements had been made for the people in hiding from the Germans for whom my mother had accepted responsibility. It was then that a scaly patch was noticed on the back of my newly born sister and the local doctor was asked for his opinion. He was not too happy about it and advised us to get a second opinion. He told Mother that he suspected it to be a kind of skin cancer. This sounded serious and yet it seemed unbelievable that such a young baby could have such a life-threatening disease.

Nowadays, I seem to come across such problems far more frequently and I am staggered to see cancer so much on the increase. The devastating effects of the disease strike at the basics of the human body, namely the cells. We see only too often that the regenerative cells are under attack, sometimes due to a poor diet, or to an enzyme deficiency or imbalance. Insufficient vitamins and minerals can also be a contributory factor, as a deficiency often means that the cells cannot function properly. We must never overlook the fact, too, that stress has a detrimental effect on our health. If I had my wish, we would never see the stress of war repeated and no doubt this goes for the majority of people who lived through those days. However, our present lives are by no means free of stress and I believe that this could have a lot of bearing on the increasing incidence of cancer. We must also ask whether our dietary habits influence our regenerative cells in a positive or negative manner. A balanced diet is an extremely important factor in the prevention and control of cancer.

Although still rather young at the time of my sister's birth, I nevertheless retain vivid memories of that period. Our general practitioner had recommended a second opinion and therefore my sister would have to be examined by a specialist at the provincial hospital. In the dark days of the war, travel was virtually impossible as there were few means of transport remaining for civilians. As our local doctor realised that speedy action was necessary, he pointed out that the best way of travelling between the hospital and our town would probably be by hearse. This vehicle was in frequent use on that stretch of road in those days, for obvious reasons. It was therefore arranged that my mother and her little daughter would be taken to and from hospital by the hearse, so that my sister could receive radium treatment.

In later years, my sister has come to realise that she made

medical history, because she was among the earliest patients to receive this kind of treatment. It was by no means a pleasant situation, but of course my mother would have done anything in her power to influence my sister's health favourably. My father had been deported by the Germans and, as a result, she had to tackle the problem virtually alone. She shouldered it courageously.

The treatment was effective, but we must remember that each cell grows, reproduces and then dies. The dead cell which has been removed must then be replaced by a new cell and here problems were encountered. As a result of the radium treatment, many of my sister's healthy cells were destroyed along with the cancerous cells and the specialist in charge of her treatment made a remark, later repeated to me by my mother, which showed a great deal of vision and insight for those days. He informed my mother that, in his opinion, the condition of her baby was the result of a one-sided food pattern – or, to put it in better English, an imbalanced diet. According to him, my sister was a product of the war, when so few foodstuffs were available. Looking back, this remark was quite revolutionary, as orthodox medicine unfortunately did not pay any attention to a possible connection between food and cancer.

Unbeknown to us at that time, this eminent specialist lived only a few minutes' walk from us. I dare say that if it was not for this gentleman, Professor A. Kolf, more kidney problems might be experienced today, because he was the inventor of the artificial kidney machine. I was very pleased when I was able to watch a film shown to the staff of a hospital I worked at, telling of how Professor Kolf had worked so hard during the war to establish the kidney machine. I only refer to this because that same eminent scientist was one of the first to recognise or even consider a possible connection between cancer and food – a very unusual viewpoint for those days.

Although my sister was finally cured of her problem, a long list of minor illnesses plagued her right up to the age of seven, from which can be deduced that the disease and its treatment took its toll on and drastically affected her immune system. Professor Kolf had warned Mother of this possibility, but he had also told her that, with luck, after the age of seven things would change for the better. In this he was also proved right. Many times I heard my mother refer to Professor Kolf with the greatest affection and admiration and, although in those days I was too young to appreciate it all, in my later studies I came to realise how ahead of his time he was.

During the war years, the medical establishment was not ready for Kolf's insistence on a balanced food pattern. Today, however, we realise more and more the probability of an inter-relationship between diet and cancer, although unfortunately the incidence of these problems is still on the increase. It is true that during the war years, particularly during the final months, there was little food to be had in terms of quantity, but it is also equally true that the available food was most likely of a better quality. Nowadays, although the required quantity is available, often the quality is lacking. Food which has been interfered with through the use of artificial fertilisers, artificial colourings, chemical additives and preservatives may carry a lot of the blame for interference with the formation of healthy cells. If the immune system, the natural defence mechanism of the body, is not able to remove the invaders of healthy cells, cancer cells can take over.

Under normal circumstances, all cellular action occurs in an orderly way. If a cell divides in order to form a new cell and no interference takes place, nothing untoward will happen. But if outside factors are allowed to interfere, a tumour may develop which could eventually turn malignant. Then other tissues may be invaded as cells travel to other parts of the body and start new growths there, and the formation of normal cells is endangered.

Nobody really knows what causes this complex disease. Modern technology and science in many fields contribute to the advance in combating certain types of cancers, but whatever is discovered often seems to increase the doubt and mystery which surrounds cancer. All discoveries concerning the possible causes of cancer are extremely useful, but it is much more essential that lessons be learned to assist us in the *prevention* of the illness. This is especially true in today's society because of the pollution of air, food and water – the three forms of energy vital to life. Elimination and prevention are of the utmost importance and therefore we should concentrate on strengthening and rebuilding the immune system, so that it is capable of withstanding attacks.

As I have said, my sister's treatment was successful. When the war ended, Mother devised a well thought out and sensible diet as soon as the situation allowed. She spared no effort in encouraging my sister's health to improve and today she is very well and the mother of two healthy sons. Occasionally when I look at her, I find it hard to believe that she once suffered the after-effects of radium treatment. By rebuilding her immune system, my sister was given the chance to develop into a healthy adult and she still follows the guidelines adhered to by our mother: a well-balanced and natural diet; no smoking or drinking. It goes to show that it is possible for people who follow a sensible diet and refrain from certain indulgences to control cancer. Moreover, I am convinced that this also goes a long way towards prevention.

I often wonder if enough investigation in this area is being carried out. Every time I come across civilisations where cancer is non-existent, it seems that they lead less stressful lives and generally follow sensibly balanced dietary patterns. Then I again recognise the wisdom hidden in the phrase, 'We are what we eat.' Environmental influence could be a possible factor in the development of cancer. Specific cancers seem to be more prevalent in certain parts of the world than elsewhere – for example:

- Liver cancer in Africa and South-East Asia
- Lung cancer in the USA and Western Europe
- Stomach cancer in Japan and Chile (probably connected with too much hot, spicy food)
- Breast cancer in Europe and the USA (could this be due to a high consumption of animal fat?)
- Cancer of the womb and the mouth and throat in India and China

Such a list leaves us wondering why these specific incidences should vary according to a seemingly geographical pattern.

It is generally believed that cancer is a disease of modern times, but in fact that is not true. In ancient Greek writings, we come across references to cancer and even in the Old Testament of the Bible diseases are referred to that sound very similar to cancer. Skeletons from ancient times discovered in Egypt show signs of tumours having formed. It is, however, a fact that cancer is becoming more prevalent. If we are to find a solution to this problem, we must leave no stone unturned in our investigations as to the cause of the illness and, better still, its prevention.

It is doubtful if allergies and viruses have ever been as prevalent as they are today. There is little doubt that viruses can be a contributory factor to cancer. When viruses are diagnosed and treated properly in their early stages, much can be done for the patient. Despite all the treatments now available in both orthodox and alternative medicine, the ones which offer the most hope are those which call upon the body's natural reserves and assist the healthy cells wherever possible to fight the abnormal cells.

Each type of cancer needs a different approach. A sarcoma – a cancer which begins in the connective tissue – will need different treatment from, for instance, a carcinoma, a cancerous growth made up of epithelial cells. A priority must be to decide on how a tumour should best be treated. It could well be the start of a neoplasm, which is an abnormal growth of tissue that can either be a benign swelling or turn out to be a malignant cancer. This malignant cancer could take the form of a carcinoma, sarcoma or leukaemia.

The lifestyle of each cancer patient should be scrutinised and he or she should be seen as a complete human being: the physical and mental aspects should both be looked at. Cancer points to the presence of disharmony and therefore every function in the body should be taken into consideration.

It is a fact that in any form of cancer, the liver – that most efficient laboratory of the body – is always involved. The liver has some dire enemies but, thank goodness, it also has a few extremely loyal friends. Nowadays, we are aware of how necessary oxygen is to the liver, assisting in the great task it performs. When the vital force in the human body is under attack, it can be aided with some of the wonderful products nature supplies to stimulate cleansing oxygen to course through the blood. It is necessary to encourage efficient blood circulation, in order that oxygen can be transported all through the body. How sad it is to see so many people endanger this function by smoking and/or drinking. We only need to look at the rise in the incidence of lung cancer to realise that one cannot get away with the statement that one's grandfather, who lived to a ripe old age, smoked most of his life. Grandfather may have been lucky, but it does not necessarily mean that his offspring is going to be equally lucky. No risks should be taken with something as vitally important as one's health.

A patient who consulted me recently wondered why he was hit by cancer because he smoked, while it had not affected his grandfather, who had lived till he was almost 90 years old and then died a peaceful death due to old age. One easily forgets that many factors play a role. I had to tell this person over and over again that his body was his own responsibility and therefore it was his duty to look after it. The quest for better health is largely a question of common sense. To encourage this gentleman, I was able to tell him that I have seen cancer that has reached even the last stage being brought back to the first stage as a result of a sensible approach.

Despite being aware that he would not like it, I advised him to give up smoking and drinking and to follow my example by drinking grape juice instead. I know that some people laugh at this, but an extremely effective method of restoring the vital force is to eat a salad of freshly grated raw beetroot, carrot and apple daily. It is generally considered too simple to be effective, but please take this advice. It was with great pleasure that I once received a letter from a young lady in which she wrote that initially she did not like the diet I had advised her to follow and most particularly disliked the beetroot I had asked her to include. However, she had read statistics about the anti-cancerous properties of beetroot and she realised that it could mean survival for her. Needless to say, she became accustomed to the taste and she was indeed rewarded because, at present, she enjoys much improved health.

For many years, I have faithfully followed the theories of my great mentor, Alfred Vogel, and I see no reason to stop now. He was a great advocate of sensible dietary management and herbal remedies to assist the lymphatic system to cleanse the liver. I have been fortunate to witness the success of this approach and am grateful for the endless studies he undertook. He closed one of his books with the advice: 'One can advise and help, but nature holds the cure. Only God the Almighty can fulfil His promise to overcome death forever.' I truly believe that if we follow the laws of nature, we obey the laws of God.

Yet have we investigated every asset available in nature? Recently, I was approached by a professor at a South African university and he pointed out that there are many plants and roots that have never been fully researched. One of these could well hold the answer to an effective cancer therapy. I am left wondering yet again why endless amounts of money have been spent on scientific research and so little effort has been made to investigate what nature may have to offer in our battle against cancer.

Let us look at cancer from another viewpoint. In 1898, *The Lancet* published an article by Dr Roger Williams in which he blamed environmental factors for the alarming increase in the death rate due to cancer in Britain. He quoted an increase from 17 to 88 people per 100,000. We must not be surprised when we hear cancer referred to as 'the disease of civilisation'.

Cancerous growths are called tumours or neoplasms and may present themselves in many ways and in different parts of the body. When found in the cells of normal tissue, the growth is called a primary tumour. This usually occurs in tissue which, in its normal function, has a constant cellular degeneration and renewal process. Most primary tumours occur at locations in which there is cell renewal due to irritation or trauma.

Primary cancers, however, rarely occur in muscle or nerve tissue, where cells do not normally subdivide or renew themselves. Liver, peritoneum, lung and bone tissue are capable of supporting the growth of a secondary tumour originating from stray cells from a primary cancer elsewhere. It is unusual to perish from a primary tumour, but whenever the cancer has metastasised, the condition is often terminal.

Metastasis – or secondary cancer – is formed of cells from the primary growths, detaching and grouping together elsewhere in the body. The circulating cancer cells do not survive. For such cells to establish a secondary growth, contact with tissue is necessary in a location which is favourable – for example, a blocked vessel, a stationary blood clot or a trauma provides a perfect place for them to settle.

When the viscosity of the blood is good and the circulation is functioning properly, the growth of the secondary cancer will be limited. Perhaps now the importance of oxygenation will be fully appreciated. The circulation of the blood can be aided by a properly balanced healthy diet and sometimes blood-thinning agents are used to obtain the right viscosity of the blood.

A specially designed diet introducing vitamins, minerals and trace elements, possibly *germanium* or *laetrile*, or some other individual remedy, may bring about a spontaneous remission from cancer. I only see recovery as feasible when the immune system can be regenerated. Stimulation of the liver function and other vital organs, together with a positive attitude by the patient, can then turn the situation around.

Some important factors in the prevention of cancer are as follows:

- Good oxygen supply
- Measures against constipation
- A good blood chemistry
- Avoidance of obesity
- Exclusion of fats, high animal protein, toxic material, nicotine and alcohol from the diet
- Avoidance, wherever possible, of stress and pollution
- Refraining from using aluminium cooking utensils
- Making sure no vitamin, mineral or trace element deficiencies exist
- Avoidance of drugs (if possible)
- Plenty of exercise in the fresh air
- Sparing use of salt

Having been in practice in Scotland for the last 35 years or so, I have seen a marked increase in bowel cancer, the rate of which is considered to be about 20 per cent higher there than elsewhere in the United Kingdom and among the highest in the world. I suppose this could be due to a higher intake of alcohol, but I have also found that a surprising number of people in Scotland suffer from constipation. Added to this, fat consumption is generally higher there than elsewhere.

We would do well to remember that the liver acts as a general detoxifier and therefore it deserves all possible help in its unique double-circulation system – the arterial blood supply and the portal blood circulation. The venous blood supply system returns the blood from the liver to the heart, whilst the portal system includes the veins, containing absorbed nutrients from the stomach. The duodenum and the small intestine drain into the large vessel known as the portal vein, which passes separately through the capillary blood vessels in the liver into general circulation. The more we encourage this process – which requires common sense more than anything else – the better we can expect our health to be. Let us not overlook the obvious: any imports must in due course be exported. It goes without saying that this ought to take place in as natural a manner as possible and without interference.

Consider the mixtures of food and drink which are often the causes of upper and lower gases, when foods ferment rather than digest: insufficient stomach acids, insufficient digestive enzymes and food soaked in alcohol all mean that it cannot be broken down into chemical compounds. These factors encourage a lack of protein-digestive enzymes and hydrochloric acid, interfering with the normal working of all those important organs.

Cancer cannot grow when the metabolism is properly balanced. As the basic unit of life lies in the cells, let us aim to stimulate the production of healthy cells. There are many ways in which the cellular system can be adversely affected. I am reminded of a young person who sought my advice after having been told that she had cancer. Fortunately, it was discovered at an early stage. After a long talk with her, I felt it necessary to perform an iridology test and a blood test. On checking the results of the iridology test, I began to wonder about the toxicity levels in her system, which indeed showed up in the blood test. I discovered that the reason for her high toxicity levels was dental amalgam, or silver mercury amalgam, so we decided to have all the amalgam removed from her dental fillings and replaced by composite fillings and an improvement was seen.

Billions of cells in our body are continuously dividing, duplicating and dying in order to maintain healthy growth, so it is quite possible that occasionally some of these cells will become faulty. Some immunologists actually believe that we produce thousands of cancer cells, but if the immune system is healthy, there is no need to worry. Seemingly minor influences, however, such as amalgam dental fillings, could play a part which should not be underestimated.

Is nature not wonderful? Think of how a baby originates – from only one cell, created by the fusion of a female ovum with male sperm! That cell multiplies to 60 trillion cells and it is reckoned that each gram of human tissue contains about 100 million cells. Consider the responsibility of looking after these healthy cells in order to keep on top of malignant cells. Nature will gratefully accept any help offered in this task!

Not so long ago, I was visited by a young man who suffered from a melanoma, a malignant neoplasm. His skin was in a dreadful condition and it is quite possible that it was caused by his working in the harsh sunshine of the Middle East. I decided on his treatment and so far the results are very encouraging. He was a sun worshipper and very proud of his tan. My advice, however, was to avoid the sun as much as possible and once I had managed to convince him, he fully cooperated. Since then, his skin has improved tremendously and it is wonderful to see how nature has restored the damaged skin, as healthy skin is beginning to reappear on the affected parts.

This process is still continuing. Often only minor adjustments are needed to effect recovery. In this case, it required some adjustment to his diet, high dosages of additional vitamin E plus vitamin C, the herbal remedies *Petasan* and *Viscasan* from Bioforce which have, as the main ingredient, *Viscum album* or mistletoe. He also took selenium and drank three glasses of raw beetroot juice daily. Many times over the years I have advised cancer patients to either drink raw beetroot juice or to eat a beetroot salad, as I described earlier. A long time ago I met a doctor in Germany who had scientifically studied the properties of beetroot. It is important that fresh, raw beetroot is used and not, as is the tendency in Britain, beetroot that has been pickled or soaked in vinegar.

As part of my training in China, I was instructed in facial diagnosis, which is widely practised there. I find myself subconsciously doing this quite frequently, as was the case when a new patient was shown into my consulting rooms. She was a lady of about 40. During our interview, I studied her closely, but I was left slightly puzzled. I could not quite make my mind up about her and therefore I decided to perform an iridology test. When studying the results of the test, I recognised signs of hereditary cancer in the areas of the liver and the pancreas. I was not completely happy about her health, either. When I asked about the medical history of her immediate relations, she told me that her mother had died of cancer of the liver and, elsewhere in the family, there had been deaths due to lung cancer and cancer of the pancreas. By no means had her condition reached an advanced stage. Iridology tests can be an extremely valuable diagnostic aid.

The Dutch alternative medicine practitioner Dr Cornelis Moerman has listed 16 clinical symptoms which may be very helpful in reaching a diagnosis. Let me state, however, that these symptoms do not automatically indicate that cancer is present, but they could serve as an early warning system if quite a few of the symptoms have been noticed. Then it is possible that a precancerous state has been reached.

1. Dryness of the skin. Excessive hard skin on the soles of the feet. Hard grains in the pores of the skin. Scaly areas on the skin. Frequently a change in the colour of the skin to a sallow complexion.
2. A change in the colour of the tongue and the inside of the lips to a deeper red.
3. Chapped skin around the corners of the mouth.
4. Scaly rings around the wings of the nose.
5. Hard and brittle nails, sometimes showing stripes on

the surface.

6. Dull hair, where a healthy gloss has disappeared.

7. Changes in the mucous membranes, noticeable with the use of a magnifying glass.

8. A certain amount of fluid retention on the inside of the lower limbs, which could also be sensitive to touch.

9. Bleeding of the gums during the brushing of teeth.

10. A marked increase in the occurrence of bruises, appearing even on light contact.

11. Slower healing process of wounds and forming of superfluous and inferior tissue in the wound.

12. Apathy, listlessness and a marked decrease in vitality.

13. Increase in inexplicable tiredness, experienced even before starting a task or activity.

14. Loss of appetite, which may result in loss of weight.

15. Blood defects such as anaemia, alkalinity or increased sedimentation.

16. General health and possible hereditary factors such as the occurrence of cancer in the family.

There are of course other ways of detecting cancer in its early stages, but great care is necessary in reaching the correct diagnosis and, to this end, blood tests are essential.

I would like to refer back to the lady whose family medical history showed various deaths due to cancer. Fortunately, in her case, we managed to detect her problems at an early stage and I prescribed *germanium* for her and a high dosage of vitamins, minerals and trace elements. I also decided on *interferon* to help her quickly.

Interferon has been of tremendous help in the treatment of certain types of cancer and is mainly obtained from leucocytes – small, colourless cells in the blood, lymph and tissues, which are important in the body's defences against infection. *Interferon* obtained from white blood cells has also proved to be effective with various cancers. Sometimes a combination of two or even three types of *interferon* is used in the more advanced cancer stages.

At times, a practitioner must have an open mind as to the treatment necessary for a particular patient. There are no hard and fast rules as to which treatment specifically combats a particular disease. Obviously there are guidelines to be followed, but the practitioner must remain flexible and at all times consider the patient as an individual and investigate his or her background.

I remember a taxi driver from the Midlands whose breathing was badly affected. I was extremely worried about him and realised that the high toxicity in his system was due to lead poisoning. It was discovered that he had cancer in a rather advanced state. To help him quickly, I used *laetrile* (also known as vitamin B17) and *germanium* (a mineral that helps neutralise harmful substances) and, on top of that, I prescribed *Ipe Roxo*, from which I think he received most benefit. *Ipe Roxo* is a herbal tea made from the inner bark of the lapacho tree from southern Brazil. Another name for this remedy is *Pau d'Arco*. Both the tea and the paste made from the bark have been used for centuries by the native Indians of Brazil for a variety of ailments, including skin cancer. About 35 years ago, it was discovered by the non-Indian community and used in the treatment of cancer when there was no other hope. Since the early '60s, the Municipal Hospital in San André has experimented with the bark in the treatment of terminal cancer patients and has reported positive results. Interestingly, it was also found that the bark cured other afflictions such as diabetes. Another of the positive effects of the tea was that it appeared to relieve the pain of the sufferers.

I also prescribed for the taxi driver *Beres* drops, a Romanian remedy rich in certain trace elements. Certain biological processes are specific in respect of their metallic ion requirements. This means that a metallic ion in a certain state is capable of taking part in the biological reactions or is able to form an adequate stereo-structure. The so-called essential elements are absolutely necessary for human and animal organisms as well as for the life of plants. Those elements which are required in small quantities only, e.g. mcg/g or less, are called trace elements. The trace elements such as copper, selenium, chromium, manganese, cobalt, etc. are suitable catalysts in enzyme reactions and have a complex relationship with hormones and vitamins. They play a role in the structural formation of bone and other tissues. In order to compensate for microelement deficiencies, or disorders due to these, *Beres* drops are prescribed since they contain those microelements which are important – according to our present knowledge – for the undisturbed function of the human body.

Not long after I first saw the taxi driver, his wife wrote to let me know that the knife-like pains in his chest had started to subside within approximately 12 hours of taking the medication. The *Beres* drops and herbal tea were beginning to bring relief. Later, he himself let me know that his specialist was very pleased to see him looking so well and that the cancer seemed to be well contained. He added that he hoped to come back and see me in a few months' time. I had also instructed him on breathing exercises and told him that controlled normal breathing was the highest form of regaining energy in the cells. This is of special importance for lung cancer patients.

This reminds me of another patient with lung cancer. She was an elderly lady who told me that she had noticed an improvement after taking ginseng. This was not surprising, as ginseng contains a lot of *germanium*, which is also the case with garlic, barley, comfrey and bitter aloe. It is very interesting to see that such energy-giving products will also help the breathing of these patients, because of the extra oxygen produced by *germanium*. I was very pleased to hear from this lady a few months later that her health was much better. Although she had previously undergone an operation on the lymph glands, this fresh outbreak of cancer after two years was now under control. Nineteen years before she had undergone a mastectomy. This lady was now able to control her cancer with dietary management backed up by several natural remedies.

There are so many methods that can be of great help. It often depends which one is suitable for the individual cancer patient, because even if there are 1,000 breast cancer patients, they will all be different and will all need an individual approach. We will look at this in Chapter Two, on breast cancer.

Chapter Two

Breast Cancer

I am very conscious of the terrible shock that women face when they suddenly discover there is something wrong with their breasts. The other day, I listened to a lady who tried to control the tone of her voice as she told me emotionally about the mastectomy she had undergone after a lump was detected in her breast. In her own words, she said, 'My breast was taken off, it was binned by the surgeon and I just had to get on with my life.' She emphasised the word 'binned', being extremely upset, although she did try to put on a brave face about her ordeal. It is quite a shock to learn that something is wrong with your body.

After seeing 13 patients with breast cancer one Saturday, I was very aware of how big this particular problem is and how many sufferers there are today. As one national newspaper reported, 'in some parts, there is an epidemic'. However, I would stress that seven out of eight breast lumps are benign and not cancerous. It is very important that a woman examines her breasts regularly, because benign breast lumps are easily treated. I often say that everybody in the world should get to know their own body, to listen to it and make sure that everything is in order, as the body will often give us warning signals if something is not right.

Breast awareness is extremely important. Not only are breasts treasured by women themselves, but also often by their partners. It is therefore important for a woman to know how her breasts look and feel normally, so that she will be able to recognise any unusual changes. It is also important to be aware of the different cycles that breasts go through – for instance, before and after a period, before and after the menopause or after a hysterectomy – and to check for any lumps, thickening or lumpiness, or nipple changes. Nipple changes – especially when the nipple becomes inverted – can be an indication of something serious and are one of the main things that will cause a doctor concern. If there is any change, one should not delay in consulting a doctor to have the cause investigated. Any change in the size or shape, any dimpling of the skin, swelling under the armpit or pain in the breast must be looked into. People are now becoming more aware of breast cancer and of the importance of self-examination. There are approximately 41,000 new cases of breast cancer diagnosed in women every year in the UK (and although very rare in men, around 300 cases are diagnosed each year). It is therefore extremely encouraging to see that screening is now routinely being carried out, as anything that can assist in the reduction of these statistics is very welcome.

I am often asked what can cause breast cancer. Although with lung cancer it is easy to say it is due to smoking, it is more difficult to say that breast cancer is triggered by any particular cause. I am aware of certain risk factors, but hormonal changes also play a big role. Genetic risk factors are possibly more common, however, and it is to one's own advantage to be observant – especially around the time of a period – of any change in the breasts, particularly with so-called cystic breasts. It is extremely important that action is taken when cysts are discovered because, although they may not cause any immediate problem, it is not advisable to leave them untreated. High dosages of vitamin C, together with the remedy *Petasites*, will very often be helpful in eliminating breast cysts. Although most are benign and not cancerous, any such cysts or lumps left untreated have the potential to become cancerous.

It is sometimes surmised that breast cancer is caused by stress and I strongly agree with this statement. As I have often said, a cancer cell is like a brain cell and stress can indeed form a precancerous situation, in which case there might be a relationship between stress and cancer. We have to deal with many emotional problems today: divorce, jealousy, work resentment, redundancies, bereavement, etc.; and it is possible that breast cancer can develop because of these additional stresses.

Sometimes women ask me if they have a greater risk of getting breast cancer because their mother or grandmother was very stressed and developed breast cancer. One could say that genes do have an influence on how susceptible we are to developing breast cancer. Therefore, if you are at all worried, it is advisable to consult a specialist for reassurance in order to allay any fears.

Breast cancer is one of the most common types of cancer in women. It accounts for approximately one in every three cases of cancer and very often occurs in slightly older women. Although it is often painless, one has to be aware of the silent situation that can manifest as a lumpy breast, small cysts or even a slight discharge from the nipple. Most tests nowadays are routinely carried out in a laboratory, where specialists can quickly establish whether there is any real cause for concern. When a specialist examines the breasts and carries out tests, such as a mammogram (an x-ray of the breasts), in most cases there is nothing to worry about.

The question, 'Can breast cancer be cured?' is often put to me. Although 'cure' is a big word, I am glad to say that I have seen many survivors and a lot of happy people who have been successfully treated using several different methods or remedies. Often women become panic-stricken when they discover some abnormality in their breasts, but the tremendous fears that they have are usually unnecessary. The vast majority of breast lumps, as I have said, are benign or harmless – that is a medical fact. Nevertheless, women should never ignore symptoms such as itching, swelling and other changes. The first thing is to keep calm, do something about it and, if there is something wrong, seek medical advice as soon as possible.

One should be aware that everybody has abnormal cells present in their body and these are mainly no cause for concern. By undergoing the breast-screening programme, one has the opportunity to investigate any problems quickly and often control the situation. Self-examination is necessary in the first instance, however – there is sufficient material available, from the NHS and other organisations, explaining the correct procedure. If any lump or other abnormality is found, you must take action quickly. It is better to be safe than sorry, but try not to become unduly alarmed. It is also very important when there is swelling or any other problem that a comfortable bra is worn – one that is not too tight.

Often when there is a breast problem and nothing else wrong, there may exist a minor lymphatic condition which can be easily assisted by lymphatic drainage (a chest lymph-drainage massage) undertaken by a qualified practitioner. The lymphatic system plays a vital role in the body by cleaning and feeding the tissues, a process which is of ultimate importance. It is very important with any breast problem – cysts, benign lumps or cancer – that the lymphatic system is cared for properly. Use only natural deodorants, take plenty of exercise, practise breathing exercises and drink sufficient still mineral water.

DAIRY PRODUCTS AND BREAST CANCER

There has recently been a lot of discussion in the press about milk. Research conducted at Oxford University into milk as a possible cause of breast cancer did not blame milk as such, but found that the insecticides, pesticides and fertilisers that are found in it may be a cause of breast cancer. In a ten-year study, it was shown that Lindane in particular has a great deal to answer for in relation to breast cancer problems. I have been working very hard to get Lindane banned for this reason.

What exactly is Lindane and why is it linked so much to breast cancer? Lindane is an organochlorine pesticide which has been used to a great extent in western Europe. For the last 60 years farmers have used it extensively. We were thankful when the relationship between Lindane and breast cancer was proved. There are serious health problems linked to this awful chemical and it also disrupts the endocrine hormonal system. Human poisoning by Lindane has been reported throughout Europe, especially in children, who are very susceptible to its toxic effects. Lindane was also noted by the International Agency for Research on Cancer and the US Environmental Protection Agency as a possible human carcinogen and an endocrine disrupter, which will affect hormones. The acceptable daily intake of its residues is very often exceeded. This pollutant is highly volatile and, when applied, the pesticide enters the atmosphere and is deposited by rain. Because it is fat soluble, it can appear in food chains and leaves its residues in the kidneys, livers and tissues – not only in humans, but also in animals.

This reminds me of a time when Dr Vogel and I conducted a lecture in Australia on the subject of DDT. We were very encouraged when a group of young people approached us after the lecture and said they wanted to spearhead a campaign to get DDT banned. It was even more encouraging when those young people eventually managed to have restrictions put on the use of DDT. As with DDT, there are many countries whose inhabitants have joined forces and established action groups to campaign for Lindane's ban. Although it is prohibited for certain uses in the United Kingdom, everyone should work extremely hard to get this powerful pesticide banned as soon as possible. We must not forget that various tests have shown the influence of Lindane on breast cancer, and it is a staggering thought that nearly 41,000 new cases of breast cancer are diagnosed every year and that one in nine women will develop breast cancer in their lifetime.

My grandmother always said that milk was 'a very peculiar lady', for when it is being produced in the body, it takes everything in that it possibly can – good or bad. It causes congestion in the system and also influences the hormonal system. Milk's good reputation is somewhat deceptive.

In the late 1960s, scientists discovered a group of proteins in breast cancer cells that could take a booster gene from the bloodstream and use it to help the cells. They called these proteins 'booster gene receptors' and there is a school of thought that a precancerous breast situation might be influenced by these particular proteins. At this point, I would like to mention that soya, although a very good product, can cause problems in breast cancer patients. It is therefore important to be careful in the use of soya in relation to the hormonal system when there is a possibility of breast cancer being present. One has to be careful with cow's milk and cheese made from it. Once hailed as a wonderful food, today cow's milk is often an enemy to many.

Milk is, strictly speaking, the only completely adequate food. Newborn children make do with it exclusively for a long period of time. From all sides, the advantages of milk are praised. Calcium, phosphorus, vitamins, protein – everything can be found in it. There is nothing wrong with this. However, whole milk has some disadvantages. To explain, I have to go back to the history of our development. For the majority of our history, we did not drink any milk, with the exception of breast-milk. When we reached adulthood there was no need to continue the production of the enzymes (mainly lactose) needed for the digestion of milk. These days, the situation has hardly changed. Most races do not have any lactose available after childhood. People from Asia and Africa do not drink milk; they cannot physically tolerate it and promptly get stomach-ache when they take it. In fact, the Chinese think a glass of milk is a terrible thing, as to them it is a glass of cow saliva!

When people who do not have enough of these enzymes drink whole cow's milk, they immediately get diarrhoea. This, however, does not apply to acid milk products. Here, bacteria have already broken down the problematic milk sugar. In Europe, especially in northern and middle Europe, we have a special situation. Those who live in the north have more lactose in their bodies. People in Scandinavia have up to 90 per cent more enzymes to break down milk sugar and therefore tolerate milk quite well. In the German-speaking countries, this percentage is much lower. Between 15 and 40 per cent of the population there do not tolerate milk. This situation is much worse in the Mediterranean countries. There, many of the population do not have the necessary enzymes for milk digestion. This north/south difference has an interesting background. The reason for it is the different grades of the sun's rays and calcium metabolism. Let me explain. An important requirement for the healthy development of bones in a child is sufficient calcium supply. As there is an abundance of calcium in plants, when a child eats sufficient vegetables, there will be no deficiency symptoms. However, the assimilation of calcium in the body is dependent on two other conditions: there should be enough vitamin D available and there should be plenty of sunlight on the skin – as here, vitamin D is changed into its usable form. In southern countries, these conditions are fulfilled and no lack of calcium is known there. In the north, the situation is different. Only in summer is there enough sunshine. Vegetables and fruit are scarce. There is a danger of lack of calcium and of rickets developing as a result. In this situation, an additional calcium supply in the form of milk is a blessing and those who can digest milk and dairy products are fortunate. During the colonisation of northern Europe, the hereditary factor of lactose was therefore a great selective advantage. Within a few thousand years, the corresponding gene spread through the people living there and the situation currently remains the same.

You will be able to tell if you have enough lactose at your disposal. When there is a marked lack of this enzyme, after drinking a glass of milk you will have excessive wind or diarrhoea. The same also applies, for example, when you eat ice cream. When there is only a slight lack of lactose, symptoms are less noticeable. Furthermore, you must realise that many foods contain milk. Therefore, stomach-aches can occur on many different occasions and this makes a clear diagnosis very difficult. Some people only find out what has been bothering them throughout their lives when they are quite old. Consequently, if you are not sure, it seems best to refrain from drinking whole milk.

Fermented or sour milk products (for example, acid milk or curd cheese) can be tolerated, as the milk sugar which causes most problems has been dealt with by bacteria. For that reason, Africans, Chinese and Indians can tolerate sour milk products quite well. Generally, the left-turning kind (L+) is best and should be favoured. Right-turning acid milk could, if used in greater quantities (more than 1 kg per day), lead to hyperacidity of the blood.

In most cases it is only necessary to avoid cow's milk – both regular and low-fat. Cream, butter and cheese are usually better tolerated: because milk sugar is soluble in water, these products contain very little of it. Acid milk products can be recommended, as they are favourable for intestinal bacteria.

Besides those with a lack of lactose, people with a tendency to allergies should be careful when considering drinking milk. You will know that some foods can provoke allergies. Milk is top of the list: 42 per cent of all food allergies are triggered by milk and it can take years or decades before this allergy is discovered in a patient.

The reason that milk is so allergy provoking comes from baby-feeding habits. After mother's milk, cow's milk is usually the first strange food that a baby comes into contact with. The intestines of a baby are different to the intestines of an adult. A baby can absorb the big protein building blocks of the milk without breaking them down first. In this way, it can extract substances that are valuable for building up the immune system from the mother's milk. However, this mechanism turns out to be very unfavourable when the baby is fed cow's milk. The protein building blocks from cow's milk are absorbed, but they are recognised as foreign matter, so the baby starts to produce antibodies against cow's milk. In certain cases, the baby can develop eczema, which comes from an inability to digest cow's milk.

It is for this reason that feeding your baby yourself is the best protection against allergies. It seems that mother's milk not only helps against food allergies, but also prevents or reduces other kinds of allergies. This is especially important when there are already other allergic tendencies in the family. If that is the case, the addition of eggs and fish to the baby's diet should be postponed as long as possible, as these foods often trigger incompatibilities.

I would like to stress something of importance here – people with stomach problems often like to drink milk, as milk binds the surplus acid. However, for a while it has been known that after binding the acids, a very high production of hydrochloric acid starts, which in its intensity is surpassed only by alcohol. The patient who is tormented by stomach-ache then starts to drink milk again, which will give relief for only a short period of time.

A person who is not allergic, has no stomach problems and does not lack lactose can drink milk without any problem. In this case, one should still remember that milk is not a drink but a meal, so one should not drink milk as a thirst-quencher between meals. A natural diet is of the utmost importance, especially in a cancer situation and also following treatment.

A survey of 1,356 naturopathic physicians in the United States and Canada has endeavoured to describe the treatments they prescribed for women with breast cancer and the perceived efficacy of their therapeutic interventions. The naturopaths were sent screening forms and a 13-page survey by investigators from Bastyr University's Cancer Research Center. The response rate was less than 50 per cent (642), which seems disappointing considering that complementary and alternative medicine use is on the rise in the United States, especially for breast cancer patients. However, it is likely that the non-respondents represent naturopathic physicians who are not involved in the treatment of breast cancer patients.

The survey results showed that 77 per cent of the respondents (497) had provided naturopathic care to women with breast cancer and 402 had treated women with breast cancer in the previous 12 months. Female naturopaths were more likely than males to treat breast cancer. Of the respondents, 6 per cent practised in the United States and 35 per cent in Canada; 66.5 per cent were women and 33.5 per cent were men.

The results showed that in developing treatment plans, naturopathic physicians most often considered the stage of cancer, the patient's emotional constitution and the conventional therapies used. To monitor patients clinically, 64 per cent used diagnostic imaging, 57 per cent considered the patient's quality of life and 51 per cent used physical examinations. The most common naturopathic therapies used were dietary counselling (94 per cent), herbal medicines (88 per cent), antioxidants (84 per cent) and supplemental nutrition (84 per cent). The most common specific treatments were vitamin C (39 per cent), coenzyme Q-10 (34 per cent) and the Hoxsey formula (29 per cent).

Naturopathy can be of tremendous help. I would stress, though, that a naturopath can only provide complementary treatment to cancer patients. By law, especially in the UK, only an oncologist is permitted to treat cancer (by the use of chemotherapy, radiotherapy, etc.), but no oncologist has a problem when a patient tries to help herself with the addition of complementary treatment, in order to rebuild her own immune system. Faced with the trauma of breast cancer, I am of the belief that there is a greater need than ever to combine the different medical approaches – at the very least, it is obvious that breast cancer requires an alternative approach to the normal, regular treatments to protect against any recurrence in the future. Chemotherapy is highly toxic and non-selective, which means that not only does it kill tumour cells but, at the same time, it also damages healthy cells. It also suppresses and damages the immune system to the extent that some patients are often left with a devastated immune system which needs further treatment.

Professor Serge Jurasunas, whom I have known for many years, gave some interesting theoretical views on breast cancer in a recent lecture. These are:

1. Breast cancer is more frequent on the left than the right side, and in the upper quadrant.
2. A determining factor may be the degeneration of surrounding mammary tissue.
3. The accumulation of food macromolecules in the extracellular environment or the cell membrane may damage cellular function and interfere with cellular communication.
4. Bacterial invasion may affect nearby solid tissue and promote malignancy or be indirectly responsible for tumour initiation.
5. Progression of a growing tumour and its sequelae depends on the interactions of malignant cells, macrophages, T-cells, mastocytes and adjacent tissue (stroma).
6. Anxiety, depressive conditions, nervous tension and social stress may be among factors associated with tumour growth.
7. Poor nutritional status, oxidative stress and inadequate antioxidants are among recognised causes of breast cancer.
8. Tobacco smoking, increased oxidative stress and lower O_2 status may induce breaks in DNA strands and initiate the tumour process.

He then gave me some very good tips on how to treat breast cancer:

1. Change your lifestyle and eating habits.
2. Seek the assistance of a certified naturopath and of a medical doctor with knowledge and experience in treating cancer.
3. Do not buy foods – especially fruit and vegetables – in large supermarkets. They are often of little nutritional value and may contain insecticides/ pesticides.
4. Visit a health food store and discover the organic foods you can include in your diet. Look for cookbooks emphasising natural eating programmes.
5. Drink at least a litre of fresh vegetable juice daily.
6. Detoxify your body and have one coffee enema per day, at least during the first month of treatment.
7. Read books on health, 'functional foods', alternative cancer methods and spiritual themes.
8. Learn how to react to chemotherapy and how to listen to your body.
9. Be patient – it takes about two years before the disease can be reversed.

When I think of the masses of patients with this problem – which is very common nowadays – I get encouragement from those who have survived. One particular lady who not only had both breasts affected by breast cancer but also her lymphatic system, told me that 28 years after being treated and by following the medical advice she was given to the letter, she never had any recurrence of her problem.

Quite a number of years ago, when I practised in the Midlands, four fairly young women came to see me one day. They had become friends with each other during chemotherapy and radiotherapy treatment at a local hospital. I saw each woman one after the other and I was happy to see how very healthy they all looked. Because of their determination to get well and, as they said, their perseverance with the 'awful' diet I gave them and the 'dreadful' glasses of beetroot juice I asked them to drink, today they are survivors and are managing to cope.

One cannot say what causes breast cancer. A young GP once came to see me. She had developed breast cancer and her lymphatic system was also under attack, in addition to other organs. She asked me if there could be any truth in what someone had told her – that she was the victim of harmful germs contracted in the infectious environment of the hospital where she worked. On the basis of scientific research, one would say no. However, because she was under very great physical and emotional stress, she believed that the cancer was a punishment for the lifestyle she led.

In former times, people believed that illness was 'a punishment of the gods' and, deep down in their hearts, many still think that. We regard illness as something bad, something which harms us and against which we have to fight with all possible means. Most people think that illness is just coincidence – bad luck – and they are convinced that bacteria and other microorganisms are to blame. Most of us think that we catch colds and other illnesses because other people contaminate us, that all kinds of germs are responsible for our disease and therefore these germs have to be destroyed with all possible means, which are provided by the pharmaceutical industry.

THE FIGHT AGAINST BACTERIA

When Louis Pasteur (1822–95) discovered that in cases of certain diseases the same bacteria were always found, he came to the logical conclusion that bacteria caused illness. For a long time, people had been looking for a scapegoat, so his discovery was received with great enthusiasm. At last the cause of all diseases had been found and now it would be possible to cure most of them. The germs only had to be killed and illness would disappear. Therefore, it was most important to find out which kind of bacteria caused each specific illness and destroy those with the right medication.

This idea worked! Thousands of patients were cured of illnesses like tuberculosis and other infectious diseases, and more children survived after serious illness. Everybody was delighted. At last, the end of all disease was near. More and more laboratories and factories, where strong medicine was produced, were built. Huge amounts of money were invested and there was work for thousands and thousands of people. Today, enormous quantities of drugs, as well as numerous new diagnostic and medical instruments and devices, are manufactured. These extremely poisonous substances are not only used in medicine, but also for agriculture and stockbreeding.

NEW DRUGS

In every respect, these new drugs were very successful, as germs were not only dangerous for people but also threatened the health and growth of fruit and vegetables, grains and cattle. Some clever and profit-conscious people even mentioned that some of these lethal drugs might be used in warfare. In short, antibiotics and other strong chemical compounds, like insecticides, herbicides and many others, were thought to be a blessing for humankind.

Were these new chemicals really such a blessing? In the beginning they most certainly were. Many patients were cured and infectious diseases lost their menace. Some of the chemicals were also a great help during operations and other interventions, as they relieved pain and prevented infection.

Nevertheless, the dream of a world without illness did not come true. Many infectious diseases could be conquered and the germs that caused them could be destroyed. However, many new diseases emerged which were hardly known before modern times. As these diseases were found mainly in the industrialised countries where the standard of living was the highest, they were called 'civilisation diseases'. Against these diseases, which spread like a forest fire, medicine seemed to be powerless.

Most of them usually started off with normal, simple health problems, which would then be treated with the same kind of medication as was used against dangerous infections. It did not seem to be important that, in this case, one 'cracked a nut with a sledgehammer'. To make symptoms disappear was the most important thing. The physician was content and the patient was happy, because the doctor had cured him or her. Apparently nobody seemed to give a thought as to how the human organism would react when symptoms were suppressed in such a drastic way.

DANGEROUS TOXINS

In our time, illness is caused mainly by toxins, poisons, unusable residues and many substances resulting from a diseased and unnatural environment. To make it easier, I will call them all 'toxins'.

Toxins are substances which get into our body through our food as well as through the respiratory tract and the skin. They also exist inside our body as metabolic waste products, morbid cells, dead bacteria, residues of cells, etc. The famous 'water doctor', Priessnitz, years ago used to describe all these toxins as 'substances that cannot be assimilated and become part of the fundamental substances of our body'. All toxins should be dissolved, be broken up and be moved to the excretive organs, where they can be disposed of.

Harmful toxins are, among others:

- The 2,500 officially registered food additives
- Chemical residues which are used in agriculture: fertilisers, insecticides, herbicides, etc.
- Many of the chemicals and synthetic drugs we use
- Harmful gases, like tobacco smoke, exhaust fumes, paint, aerosol sprays, etc.
- Deodorants, vaginal sprays, different perfumes, cosmetics, washing and cleaning substances, soap, etc.

Such toxins, which are foreign substances to our organism and have no business being there, get into the body by way of the intestines, the lungs, the skin and the mucous membranes, and eventually accumulate in all body tissues. They can also damage our vital organs. For our body, dealing with such foreign matter is not a natural task. Our defensive mechanisms are constantly overtaxed. Many toxins originate in the organism itself and come especially from the polluted contents of our intestines.

DISEASE-PROVOKING INFLUENCES

Apart from germs, the causes of illness are most often:

- Wrong eating habits
- Too little sleep or sleeping at the wrong time
- Great changes in temperature
- Emotional problems or too much stress
- Too little exercise
- Lack of fresh air and oxygen
- Lack of light and sunlight

Generally, there is far too little elimination of toxins and, as a consequence, there is often a dangerous accumulation of waste products in the body.

Of course, we know that genetic factors can also contribute to the development of disease, but when healthy eating habits and the other guidelines mentioned above are generally adhered to negative genetic factors often stay dormant and do no harm. The reasons for illness mentioned above are basically the same as in the past. However, today the dangers to our health are far more threatening.

Most of the disease-provoking factors mentioned above speak for themselves. However, due to our modern lifestyle, sexual problems also play an important role in the development of disease and we should remember how important it is to practise safe sex.

Going back to the young GP who consulted me about her cancer, I told her that as she herself knew only too well, cancer was not infectious, but that toxic substances might have had some influence. Both internal and external influences have a damaging effect. Toxicity, stress and emotional problems all play a part in the development of cancer. According to Dr Hans Selye, we all need a measure of stress. Normal stress is a challenge and strengthens the body's defences. However, abnormal and excessive stress, from which millions of people in the industrial countries suffer, can overtax us physically as well as mentally.

The natural balance is being destroyed. Health and illness are based on very specific natural laws, which must always be observed. These laws concern the constant changes of being awake and asleep, day and night, work and relaxation, happiness and sadness, and so on. Formerly, people were obliged to go to bed early and to rise early. In those times, daily life depended on daylight and candles were expensive. Nowadays, there are many people who do not go to sleep before midnight and even later. As our organism still reacts to natural sources of light, this habit usually has a negative effect on our nervous system.

MONEY AND POSSESSIONS
In the industrial countries, there are millions of people who only work in order to earn the money they need for their livelihood; they do not care for the work as such. This can be considered as a very negative stress factor. Unfortunately, although most people now earn much more than ever before, this does not improve their health.

Apart from normal daily expenses, what do people do with their money? They often buy things they like, but do not really need. By gathering possessions, they try to build up their 'image'. This means they want to impress on their friends and neighbours that they are doing well, according to the principle that people who have many possessions are clever and should be admired.

The more primitive a person is, the more he or she wants to possess and to buy. He therefore always needs more money and has to work harder. In this way, countless people get into an unnecessary and constantly stressful situation.

As I said earlier, stress can overtax us, both physically and mentally. I saw this clearly with one of my assistants, who had a very successful mastectomy. I treated her afterwards and everything was fine until she discovered that her husband was having an affair with his secretary. She was devastated and could not come to terms with what had happened. Sadly, it ended in divorce. She then developed ovarian cancer. Luckily, with a lot of work and effort, we were able to control this and she is now well.

I do think it is necessary, as one of my recovered patients said, for one to follow one's practitioner's instructions to the letter in order to overcome this monstrous problem. This means not only sticking to good dietary management, but also taking the recommended remedies and carrying out proper breathing exercises, positive visualisation and meditation.

Chapter Three

Breast Cancer and HRT

As I have said for many years in lectures, hormone replacement therapy has many benefits. I would be dishonest if I said I have never prescribed or recommended its use. Over the years I have been in practice, women have almost attacked me when I have suggested it was time they came off HRT and I have frequently heard them say what a change HRT has brought to their lives. Without doubt, HRT does a lot of good – not only for menopausal symptoms, but also when there is a decline or a complete cessation of oestrogen production by the ovaries. In many cases, oestrogen deficiency leads to a number of short- and long-term physical and psychological symptoms that can often be prevented. As we all know, HRT helps replace the body's hormonal oestrogen. We hear repeatedly that in order to control hot flushes and, as one gets older, osteoporosis, HRT is the only answer. Stress factors often play a role in premenstrual and premenopausal problems, giving all kinds of distressing symptoms such as dryness or narrowing of the vagina, which often makes intercourse difficult or impossible. The stress that this brings on could affect the heart and, especially in menopausal women, hypertension or diabetes often results. Sadly, these conditions are regularly left untreated as women either believe that they will go away in their own good time, or they don't want any interference; they are embarrassed or their doctors are unsympathetic. The underlying cause – especially with menopausal problems – should be recognised and when the symptoms are alleviated, the associated anxieties frequently disappear.

As there are many natural alternatives available today, any synthetic remedies should be taken with care and used only when necessary. Oral oestrogen replacement is not often necessary but can sometimes, if well controlled, be very effective. One should never forget the risks of HRT – carcinoma of the womb is one. The breasts may also be oestrogen-sensitive and any carcinoma will grow very much faster with the use of this hormone, so women who have tumours or fibroids are usually advised against taking HRT. One should also be very careful when there is heart disease present. I repeat that, although this treatment might be effective, you should use your common sense (there is nothing common about common sense!) and try the natural alternatives in the first instance. Oral oestrogen replacements are easier than oestrogen absorption through the skin with the use of HRT patches, but both should be monitored very carefully.

There is no doubt that HRT has many benefits – it will prevent osteoporosis, as well as possibly strokes and heart disease – but there are always risks when taking an artificial substance. In the 48 years that I have been in practice, I have seen the after-effects of HRT many times – not only phlebitis and thrombosis, but also breast cancer. I promised myself some time ago that I would warn people – which I also do on radio and television – to ensure that mistakes are not made. Granted, the recent scares regarding the use of HRT have probably been exaggerated and the negative side of HRT has been magnified beyond belief.

If you have the slightest worry over breast swelling, enlarged lymph glands or a change in size or shape, changes in the skin, thickening or lumps, or bloodstained discharge from the nipples, you should have the problem investigated. It is particularly important with breast cancer (the commonest form of female cancer) to be vigilant. The huge number of women who die every year of the disease is very worrying indeed. The increased incidence of breast cancer due to the use of HRT is evident, however controversial it is. For those who decide to take HRT, a wholesome diet is very important, with plenty of fruit and vegetables, and the inclusion of vitamins A, E and C, to help maintain a normal healthy lifestyle. Taking a gentle approach is important when HRT is involved.

Relaxation techniques and stress management, in combination with recommended remedies, are both physically and emotionally helpful. When a woman discovers she has a disease like cancer, severe depression can set in, which can become very debilitating and often the patient will need extra medical help in lifting this depression. The inclusion of acupuncture, homoeopathic remedies and breathing exercises can be beneficial. I often find cranial osteopathy (which will greatly help the endocrine and lymphatic systems) to be extremely helpful with such conditions.

It is frightening enough to discover a lump in the breast, but when told it is cancerous, we see the terrible panic women face, which is completely understandable. To help women over this initial shock, I have found an old herbal remedy made many years ago by the herbalist Charlie Abbott, *Composition 3* (half a teaspoonful, taken twice a day), to be of benefit.

A young female patient once consulted me because she felt extremely tired, had no appetite and was listless and emotional. When I looked at her, I could see that her lymphatic system was causing problems. I asked her if she self-examined her breasts and she told me that she noticed one of her nipples was becoming inverted. She had pain, not only under her arms, but also between her legs and in her neck – all areas where we have lymph glands. As soon as I realised this, I asked her to go and see her doctor so that she could be checked properly.

Nowadays, with so much stress and worry as part of our daily lives, it is very important that we take care of our lymphatic system. Every day I see many patients who are the victims of breast cancer. The lymph glands, which work through the night by cleansing the waste material that the body gathers during the day, are often overworked. Whenever there is toxicity in the blood or one feels unwell and a precancerous situation occurs, the alarm bells of the lymphatic system start ringing. With HRT-dependent women, there can be a high level of toxicity present and this can trigger the development of a precancerous condition.

The daily intake of vitamins, minerals and other recommended supplements, either on their own or in combination, is very important. One supplement whose efficacy has been demonstrated in preventing cancer and boosting the immune function is *IP-6* combined with *inositol*, which has been researched and patented by Professor A. Shamsuddin. *IP-6* comes from the bran portion of brown rice.

The lymphatic system – the white bloodstream – is crucially important to our health, but our knowledge of it is still very limited. The lymphatic vessels, which are much finer and longer than those of the red bloodstream, are distributed throughout the entire body. In contrast to the blood, the lymph flows only in one direction and the fluid is returned to the bloodstream after its task is completed. The body can be divided schematically into four parts in the form of a cross, starting at the navel. Each of these four fields more or less corresponds to a lymphatic network, with a centre located at the right and left side of the groin area and in each of the armpits. Smaller centres are also located below the lower jaw at the right and left side. Leading to these centres, the lymph glands form little nodes, which reach their maximum size in the centre itself.

FUNCTIONS OF THE LYMPHATIC SYSTEM

The lymphatic system is responsible for keeping the body fluids, the blood and the cerebrospinal fluid in order. The total amount of fluid accounts for approximately 60 per cent of our total body weight. But the lymph has yet another important and vital function. Not unlike a police force, the lymph cells (lymphocytes, also called phagocytes and wandering cells) must combat and destroy all invading organisms that enter and endanger the body tissue. I am referring to bacteria, which are more or less injurious and dangerous, depending on the type. For example, if you cut yourself or a rusty nail penetrates the skin, millions of bacteria advance into the nodes of a centre, then call up the defences; the vessels expand and we feel a swelling in the area of the armpit or the groin, for example. The swelling can become as large as a hen's egg. If the lymphocytes cannot handle their task, the lymphatics become inflamed and swollen. They become sensitive to pressure and can be seen as red lines. This condition is called blood poisoning (septicaemia, toxaemia), even though the toxins are actually still contained in the white bloodstream of the lymphatic system. In fact, if all toxins and bacteria were passed on to the red bloodstream, no one would survive childhood because of the many poisons that would enter the blood in that time.

In the event that cancer cells escape during a biopsy or because of incomplete removal of malignant tissue in the operation, the lymph generally catches them and the centre harbours them with the intention of destroying them. If the attempt to destroy them fails, these giant cells begin to grow and multiply, and the result is the much-feared lymphoadenoma, or Hodgkin's disease, a form of cancer of the lymph nodes. That is why surgeons remove lymphatic vessels and nodes during a cancer operation, especially in breast cancer.

SAGE (*SALVIA OFFICINALIS*)
Without doubt, oestrogen supplementation was a tremendous finding, but we have natural remedies without any side effects which are very helpful – such as the herb *Salvia officinalis* (sage). This herb almost shouts out what it should be used for, as it gets specks of perspiration on its leaves when the sun shines – in other words, the plant has a signature characteristic which tells us that when we get hot and bothered, as very often menstrual and menopausal women do, there is a plant here in nature which will not only help these conditions but could also prevent a precancerous situation developing.

MENOSAN
Application
Hot flushes, excessive sweating, excessive salivation and inflammation/ulceration of mouth and throat.

The menopause signals the beginning of a new stage in a woman's life. This usually occurs between the ages of 45 and 60, although it may start in the mid- to late 30s. Menopause is a time of fundamental hormonal and functional adjustment, and many of the distressing symptoms such as hot flushes, mood changes, insomnia, palpitations, vaginal soreness and cystitis are a result of the body trying to adapt to these changes. *Salvia officinalis* (sage) is a phyto-oestrogen but does not contain any oestrogenic molecules. Its action depends on the ability to trigger oestrogen production by oestrogen-producing cells and its oestrogenic effects when binding to oestrogen receptors. Its direct antibacterial action is useful for inflammation of the mouth and throat when related to infections.

Description

Menosan is prepared from the fresh leaves of *Salvia*. *Salvia* is a mild phyto-oestrogen. Phyto-oestrogens are defined as substances which possess the potential of influencing oestrogenic activity in the body to varying degrees. These substances bind to oestrogen receptor sites of cells, triggering oestrogenic activity. *Salvia* is one of our oldest medicinal plants. The Greeks and Romans first used it as a preservative for meat. It was believed that, amongst other things, it could improve the memory and increase wisdom – which probably gave us the origin of the herb's common name, sage. This has greater relevance in that the herb has been investigated for its use in Alzheimer's disease. *Salvia* contains volatile oils, tannins and flavonoids. In the past, it has been used for a wide variety of conditions. Nowadays its prime role is as a useful remedy for alleviating excessive sweating and menopausal hot flushes.

Mode of Action

> Phyto-oestrogen
> Oestrogenic action
> Hypothalamic action
> Antiseptic
> Astringent

Around the time of menopause, the amount of oestrogen produced by the ovaries begins to diminish. The lower levels of hormones in the blood trigger the release of a specific regulating factor from the hypothalamus in the brain, encouraging more hormone production from the ovaries. The hypothalamus is also the control centre for temperature regulation. It is an important intermediary between the nervous system and the endocrine system. Many of the physical and mental symptoms which occur during menopause are a result of an imbalance in this control mechanism. *Salvia* has a rebalancing effect on the hypothalamus, correcting sweat regulation. Taken internally, it can reduce the secretion of saliva. The volatile oils (especially thujone) in *Salvia* are antiseptics. Tannins are anti-inflammatory and astringent, and this combination is useful for throat and mouth infections and inflammation, especially when used as a gargle.

Dosage
Fifteen to twenty drops, three times a day before meals, in a little water. If night sweats are particularly severe, thirty drops should be taken before bedtime. As a gargle: ten drops in half a cup of hot water to be used four to six times a day as needed, for sore throats.

Duration of Administration
No restrictions to long-term use.

Restrictions
Those who suffer from diabetes and epilepsy should consult a healthcare professional before using *Menosan*. Do not take in combination with Tamoxifen. This product is not recommended during pregnancy and nursing unless directed by a healthcare professional.

Ingredients
Fresh plant tincture (100 g) typically contains the tincture of:
Salvia officinalis (sage) 100 g
(Alcohol content: approximately 66 per cent)

BLACK COHOSH (CIMICIFUGA RACEMOSA)
Another marvellous remedy is *Black Cohosh*, a herb which is used particularly for menstrual and menopausal problems.

Application

Dysmenorrhoea, menopausal symptoms and premenstrual syndrome (PMS).

Two types of dysmenorrhoea (painful periods) can affect women. Primary (spasmodic) dysmenorrhoea is experienced in younger women. It is caused by the uncoordinated uterine contractions which occur at the start of a period. This produces a colic-type pain in the lower abdomen, back and legs, which can last for up to 48 hours. Secondary (congestive) dysmenorrhoea occurs more often in older women. It may be caused by factors such as pelvic inflammatory disease, pelvic congestion, endometriosis, pelvic adhesions or fibroids. The pain starts as a dull ache in the lower abdomen or lower back.

Black Cohosh is particularly effective at easing uterine cramps. It alters the oestrogen/progesterone balance in favour of oestrogen. This makes it useful for menopausal and menstrual problems associated with depression, where a dominance of progesterone is believed to play a part.

Description

A fresh herbal extract of the root of *Black Cohosh*. It is a member of the buttercup family and was originally used by the native American Indians for its 'normalising' and relaxant effects on the female reproductive system. In modern phytotherapy, *Black Cohosh* is used particularly for painful periods and problems associated with the menopause.

Mode of Action

> Oestrogen-like action
> Reduction in luteinising hormone (LH) release from the
> pituitary gland

Black Cohosh contains several important constituents – triterpene glycosides (actein, cimicifugoside), isoflavones (formononetin) and salicylic acid. Triterpene glycosides such as cimicifugoside have an effect on the hypothalamus-pituitary system, reducing the concentration of LH. This, in turn, decreases progesterone production from the ovaries. Formononetin has been found to act on oestrogen receptors, but it does not reduce serum LH levels. Clinical trials have shown that *Black Cohosh* is useful for hot flushes and the emotional problems associated with the menopause which would normally benefit from HRT. The mode of action of *Black Cohosh* in the treatment of menstrual difficulties is not clear. It seems to act both directly on the tissues of the reproductive system and indirectly through the hypotensive, vasodilatory and anti-inflammatory activity. Actein, one of the triterpene glycosides, causes peripheral vasodilation and an increase in peripheral blood flow. *Black Cohosh* contains a natural source of salicylic acid, which has an anti-inflammatory and mild analgesic action in painful inflammatory conditions.

Dosage Information
Fifteen to twenty drops twice a day, in a little water.
Maintenance: twenty drops once a day, in a little water.

Duration of Administration
If *Black Cohosh* is needed long term, it is recommended that a one-month break from treatment is taken after six months.

Restrictions
If on the birth control pill or HRT, use only under the direction of a healthcare professional. Gastrointestinal disturbances are occasionally experienced. Should not be taken by those allergic to aspirin. It is not recommended during pregnancy or nursing unless directed by a healthcare professional.

Ingredients
Fresh plant tincture (100 g) typically contains the tincture of:
Black Cohosh (*Cimicifuga racemosa*) 100 g
(Alcohol content: approximately 65 per cent)

FEMALE ESSENCE
Alternatively, one could try *Female Essence*, which is a flower remedy and, again, is of tremendous benefit. It helps maintain a

feeling of emotional balance and well-being in women. Not only is it particularly helpful around the time of the period, but it also helps menopausal symptoms, sexual problems and infertility, stress and fatigue.

Dosage
Five drops in a little water, three times daily, starting before symptoms arise. If particularly stressed, use at intervals up to six times daily.

Another option would be to try a combination of vitamins, minerals and trace elements, such as *Female Balance, Menopause Factors, Healthy Cells™ Breast* and *Phytogen* (a marvellous product).

Ingredients
Olive: for extreme tiredness and exhaustion, a common symptom of PMS. Brings strength

Cherry Plum: for tension headaches, out-of-control feelings, inability to cope and anxiety. Brings calm and ease

Crab Apple: physical cleansing assists correct menstrual flow and helpful for water retention. Helps a woman feel comfortable about her bodily functions

Pomegranate: the primary remedy for women. Can be helpful for all female physical problems, enhancing feelings of security and nurturing and acceptance of one's femininity

Copper Beech: for the vagueness so common during PMS. Clearing and energising. Brings feelings of space around you with security and grounding

Walnut: gives protection at this vulnerable time, also regulates hormonal balance

Water Violet: during the menstrual cycle, there is a need to seek personal space, which may prove difficult with the demands of a busy life. Helps one to keep a sense of inner space whilst staying comfortably connected to others

Scleranthus: for mood swings, clumsiness and indecisiveness, common symptoms of PMS. Helps one stay centred

Morning Glory: reduces the need for stimulants such as caffeine and sugar, another common symptom of PMS

Impatiens reduces feelings of irritation and impatience. Also for period pains. Brings patience, calm and understanding

FEMALE BALANCE

Female Balance provides essential vitamins and minerals that are depleted in women who experience premenstrual syndrome (PMS). These critical nutrients are combined with concentrated extracts of herbs that women have depended on for centuries. *Female Balance* was formulated exclusively for Enzymatic Therapy by my son-in-law and myself.

Dosage
Three to six capsules daily during periods of PMS as an addition to the everyday diet.

Ingredients
Essential vitamins and minerals:
Vitamin A (Beta-carotene) (non-toxic form of vitamin A) 16,665 iu
Vitamin E (D-Alpha tocopherol succinate) 200 iu
Vitamin C (Ascorbic acid) 200 mg
Magnesium L-Aspartate 150 mg
Pantothenic Acid (D-Calcium pantothenate) 100 mg
Thiamine HCL (Vitamin B1) 50 mg
Riboflavin (Vitamin B2) 50 mg
Calcium Citrate 50 mg
Iron (Ferrous succinate) 18 mg
Zinc (Gluconate) 15 mg
Chromium (Polynicotinate) 250 mcg
Folic Acid 100 mcg
Vitamin B12 (Cyanocobalamin concentrate) 50 mcg
Selenium (L-Selenomethionine) 50 mcg

Other ingredients:
Dong Quai extract (4:1) (Angelica sinensis) 75 mg
Liquorice Root extract (Glycyrrhiza glabra) – standardised to contain 5 per cent glycyrrhizic acid 60 mg

OK OK

FEMALE CANCERS

Milk Thistle extract (Silybum marianum) – standardised to contain 70 per cent silymarin calculated as silybin 50 mg
Black Cohosh extract (4:1) (Cimicifuga racemosa) 30 mg
Chaste Berry extract (5:1) (Vitex agnus-castus) 20 mg
Pyridoxal-5'-Phosphate 10 mg

Contains no sugar, salt, yeast, wheat, corn, dairy products, colouring, flavouring or preservatives.

MENOPAUSE FACTORS
This is another wonderful remedy.

Ingredients
Vitamin C: essential for the growth and repair of tissues in all parts of the body. Plays a vital role in the health of the immune system
Vitamin E: useful in alleviating symptoms associated with the menopause and has been used for the incidence of hot flushes
Vitamin B6: essential for the metabolism of essential fatty acids and amino acids. Necessary for the health of the nervous system, the immune system and the skin
Pantothenic Acid: supports the function of the adrenal glands and necessary for the metabolism
Calcium Chelate: an easily absorbable form of calcium, essential for bone health and aids production of energy
Iodine: required by the thyroid gland and controls the metabolic rate
Magnesium: plays an essential role in maintaining the health of the bones
Borage: acts as a restorative agent on the adrenal glands
Dong Quai Root: beneficial in treating muscle cramps and pain associated with painful periods
Mexican Wild Yam Root: valuable in relieving ovarian and uterine pains
Liquorice Root: has a balancing effect on hormones and soothes inflamed mucous membranes, as well as stimulating the action of the adrenal glands

Black Cohosh Root: relieves menstrual cramps and depression, as well as hot flushes and vaginal atrophy. Beneficial in alleviating emotional symptoms associated with the menopause, due to its action of balancing and regaining normal hormonal activity

Passion Flower: has a soothing effect on the nerves and is also useful as an anti-spasmodic

Red Clover: this plant contains all four of the important isoflavones that have been identified to be the protective components of traditional diets commonly associated with reduced menopausal complications

HEALTHY CELLS™ BREAST

Breast health is one of the most important issues to women of all ages. *Healthy Cells™ Breast* contains vitamins, minerals and herbs which clinical studies have shown help develop and maintain healthy breast cells.

How Does It Work?

Metabolism of active foreign substances, or detoxification, is a process that requires enzymes. The enzymes involved in detoxification are generally divided into two groups, known as Phase I and Phase II enzymes. Phase I enzymes, such as cytochrome P450-dependent monooxygenase, convert hydrophobic (fat-soluble) compounds to electrophilic (active) derivatives. Phase II enzymes, which include glutathione transferase, glucuronosyltransferase and sulfotransferase catalyse conjugation reactions. Most reactions catalysed by Phase II enzymes produce high polar molecules that are readily excreted from the body. While the Phase I reactions tend to be an activating process, the Phase II reaction is more likely to be a detoxification process.

Glucuronidation is a major pathway to the Phase II detoxification process. It is catalysed by glucuronosyltransferase and requires the co-factor UDP-glucuronic acid. When glucuronidated, these compounds become polar, water-soluble conjugates that are eliminated from the body in urine and bile. However, active compounds conjugated with glucuronic acid are substrates of b-glucuronidase. B-glucuronidase can reconvert substances back to their Phase I, potentially harmful form, which reabsorbs into the body and delays the elimination of these compounds.

Calcium D-Glucarate

Calcium D-glucarate (CGT) is a precursor of glucarolactone (GL), which inhibits b-glucuronidase. By inhibition of b-glucuronidase, GL increases the amount of these compounds sequestered and excreted as the glucuronides, thus decreasing the portion of active compounds that could be hazardous to the body. In animal studies, administration of CGT was reported to inhibit b-glucuronidase activity. CGT was also found to support healthy cell development.

Increased clearance of endogenous estradiol and precursors of 17-ketosteroids, followed by the reduction in steady-state levels of these hormones, are theorised as further explanation for this supplement's support of healthy breast cells.

Folic Acid

Folic acid functions as a carrier of hydroxymethyl and foryl groups. Folic acid is necessary for the synthesis of purine and thymine, required for the formation of DNA, thus making it essential for cell growth and reproduction. Folic acid is required for red blood cell maturation. Additionally, a study demonstrated that folic acid supports breast health in women who also consume alcohol.

Vitamin B12

Vitamin B12 performs several metabolic functions. Acting as a coenzyme, vitamin B12 is necessary for red blood cell formation and maturation, amino acid and fatty acid metabolism. A study has suggested that vitamin B12 deficiency may lead to reduced DNA synthesis and impaired DNA repair mechanism in breast tissue in the lab setting. Both of these mechanisms are required for healthy cells.

Protein-Bound Iodine

Protein-bound iodine is involved in making thyroid hormones, which help regulate reproduction, maintenance of healthy metabolic rates, and cell growth. Clinical studies have demonstrated that iodine is essential for breast health. The effects of iodine on breast tissue are thought to render intralobular duct cells less sensitive to circulating oestrogens.

Broccoli
Broccoli is a vegetable from the genus *Brassica*. It contains a large number of phytochemicals, some of which have been shown to be beneficial to preventing breast cancer. In the early 1900s, broccoli was found to increase the activity of Phase II enzymes. Later, sulforaphane was identified as the principal Phase II enzyme in broccoli extract. In animal studies, sulforaphane was reported to enhance chemical detoxification and support healthy cell development.

Green Tea
Green tea is a dried product of the fresh shoot of the tea plant (*Camellia sinensis*) from which numerous biological activities have been reported. A 1998 study indicated that green tea supports breast health in a variety of ways. Green tea is a rich source of flavonoids and polyphenols, namely catechins and flavonols. The catechins, also known as tea polyphenols, which occur in significant quantities in green tea, are catechin, epicatechin, gallocatechin, epigallocatechin, epicatechin gallate and epigallocatechin gallate (EGCG). A study has indicated that EGCG supports healthy breast cell development.

Maitake D-Fraction Compound
Maitake mushroom (*Grifola frondosa*) is an edible mushroom consumed in China and Japan, both for its taste and health benefits. Recently, its powder and water extracts have been investigated for effects on the immune system and support of healthy cell development. Maitake D-fraction is a mixture of b-D-glucan fraction obtained from Maitake water extracts. It mainly contains b-1,6' D-glutan with b-1,3' branches. In an animal model, D-fraction was shown to activate macrophages, natural killer cells and cytotoxic T-cells with a concomitant increase in interleukin-1

production. In the spring of 1998, an investigational new drug application was obtained from the Food and Drug Administration (FDA) for the use of D-fraction in a Phase II pilot study.

TABLE 2: POSSIBLE MECHANISMS OF ACTIONS FOR INGREDIENTS IN *HEALTHY CELLS*™ *BREAST*

Ingredient	Functions
Calcium	● D-glucarate inhibits b-glucuronidase activity
	● Increases glucuronidation and detoxification
	● Increases clearance of oestrogens
	● Supports healthy cell development
Broccoli concentrate	● Induces the activity of Phase II enzymes
	● Stimulation of detoxification systems
	● Supports healthy cell development
Green tea extract	● Antioxidant and free-radical scavenging activity
	● Stimulation of detoxification systems
	● Supports healthy cell development
Maitake powder/ D-fraction	● Activates macrophages, natural killer cells and cytotoxic T-cells
	● Increases interleukin-1 production
	● Supports healthy cell development
Folic acid	● Essential for cell growth and reproduction
	● Supports red blood cell maturation
	● Adequate folic acid intake is supportive to breast health
Vitamin B12	● Coenzyme necessary for red blood cell formation, amino acid and fatty acid metabolism
	● Adequate vitamin B12 is supportive to DNA synthesis, cell growth and development

Iodine	● Involved in making thyroid hormones, which help to regulate reproduction and cell growth
	● Makes interlobular duct cells less sensitive to circulating oestrogen
	● Essential for breast health

Dosage
One tablet, twice daily, with meals.

Ingredients
Folic Acid 200 mcg
Vitamin B12 (as cyanocobalamin) 500 mcg
Calcium D-glucarate (provides 25 mg of elemental calcium) (D-Glucarate™ brand) 200 mg
Iodine (from casein iodide) 212.5 mcg
Broccoli (*Brassica oleracea*) floret and stalk concentrate standardised to contain a minimum of 125 mcg sulforaphane 125 mg
Green Tea (*Camellia sinensis*) leaf extract (decaffeinated) standardised to contain a minimum of 70 per cent polyphenols 50 mg
Maitake (*Grifola frondosa*) mushroom powder 50 mg
Maitake (*Grifola frondosa*) mushroom extract standardised to contain a minimum of 28 per cent D-fraction compound 5 mg

Other ingredients:
Cellulose, modified cellulose gum, stearic acid, silicon dioxide, magnesium stearate and titanium dioxide colour

Contains no sugar, salt, yeast, wheat, gluten, corn, soy, artificial flavouring or preservatives. All colours used are from natural sources.

THE FEMALE BREAST
The female breast is a complex structure of variable size, consistency and composition. Although anatomically distinct, the

breasts are functionally related to the female genitourinary system in that they respond to cyclic changes in sex hormones and produce milk for infant nourishment. Breast tissue changes throughout the life cycle: in puberty as the female breasts develop and sexual maturation begins; during pregnancy in preparation for lactation; after childbirth in milk production; and during menopause and later life with replacement of glandular (functional) tissue with adipose (fat) tissue.

Structurally, the breast consists of fibrous connective tissue, fat and glandular tissue. The superficial (upper layer) connective tissue of the breast is attached to the skin. Muscles and fibrous connective tissue support the breast mass itself. Cooper's ligaments provide additional support to the breast and divide the breast into 15 to 25 lobes, similar to spokes on a wheel. Each lobe consists of mammary glands or alveoli, grape-like structures that are lined with secretory cells capable of producing milk. The glands are connected by a series of ducts, which transport milk from the glands to the nipple. The nipple is located centrally on the breast and is surrounded by the pigmented areola.

Effects of Hormones on the Breast
Oestrogen initiates growth of the breasts and of the milk-producing apparatus. It is also responsible for the characteristic external appearance of the mature female breast.

Progesterone promotes development of the lobules and glands of the breasts, causing the glandular cells to proliferate, enlarge and become secretory in nature. However, milk is only secreted after the hormonally prepared breast is further stimulated by the pituitary hormone prolactin. Progesterone causes the breasts to swell. Part of this swelling is due to the secretory development in the lobules and alveoli, but partly also results from increased fluid in the subcutaneous (below the skin) tissue.

The hormonal influence on breast cancer is well demonstrated, in that gender is the most significant risk factor for the development of the disease. Women develop breast cancer 100 times more frequently than men. While hormones themselves are not carcinogenic, prolonged exposure to oestrogen and progesterone are associated with increased cancer incidence. Early onset of menses, late menopause, and late first pregnancy or no history of pregnancy are linked to exposure to hormones that may have a significant role in the development of breast cancer.

Changes in the Breast during the Menstrual Cycle
Fluid is produced and reabsorbed during the female menstrual cycle. The breasts respond to cyclic changes in the menstrual cycle with fullness and discomfort.

Changes in the Breast with Pregnancy
Significant changes occur in the breast during pregnancy. In response to hormones, the ducts and alveoli increase in number and size. This causes the breast to enlarge to two or three times their pre-pregnancy size. Breast milk is produced in response to complex hormonal changes associated with pregnancy.

Changes in the Breast with Menopause
With the onset of the menopause, oestrogen and progesterone levels gradually decline. There is a gradual decrease in glandular tissue. Decomposition of the lobes and alveoli begins. After menopause, glandular tissue continues to decompose and is replaced by fat. The breasts tend to hang more loosely from the chest wall because of these tissue changes and the relaxation of Cooper's ligaments.

Fibrocystic Changes
Fibrocystic changes are a result of the formation of benign (non-cancerous) cysts along the ducts. These cysts are filled with fluid and are usually noted in both breasts. The cysts are tender and painful, especially premenstrually. In the past, fibrocystic changes were referred to as 'fibrocystic disease'. Because this condition affects at least half of all women at some point in their lives, it is more accurately defined as a change rather than as a disease. Fibrocystic changes are most common in women between 35 and 50, but can affect women of any age.

FEMALE CANCERS

Fibroadenomas

Fibroadenomas are benign (non-cancerous) tumours made up of both glandular breast tissue and fibroconnective (supporting) tissue. They most often occur in both breasts. They are most common in young women in their 20s and 30s, although they may occur at any age. Fibroadenomas generally do not cause pain or tenderness and do not respond to hormonal influences of the menstrual cycle. Some fibroadenomas are quite small, while some may be several inches in size. They tend to be round and have borders that are distinct from the surrounding breast tissue. They are well delineated and mobile when palpated, so they often feel like a marble within the breast.

Breast Cancer

As I have said earlier, cancer of the breast is the most common cancer in females. One in eight women will have breast cancer in her lifetime. Peak incidence of malignancy is between the ages of 40 and 60, with two-thirds of malignant breast tumours occurring in women under 65. In about 80 per cent of women with breast cancer, a painless lump is the initial symptom. Malignant tumours generally occur in only one breast and are most often a single mass, irregular in shape and hard and stone-like. The tumour does not move upon touching or pressing with the hand, and is generally not tender, with poorly delineated and irregular borders. Malignant tumours do not vary with the menstrual cycle. Breast cancer can occur within the ducts, in the lobes, or in the basic tissue of the breast itself. Breast cancer occurs more frequently in the left breast than in the right and more often in the upper outer quadrant.

PHYTOGEN

An estimated three million women in the UK are between the ages of 45 and 55 – the stage in life when the menopause is most likely to occur. At this age, women's bodies begin to produce less oestrogen, triggering the onset of the menopause and often a number of distressing symptoms such as hot flushes, irregular bleeding and mood swings. Symptoms can last from two to five years. There are also silent conditions that include high blood cholesterol, high blood pressure and osteoporosis.

As we have seen, the most popular treatment choice for menopausal symptoms is synthetic oestrogens in the form of HRT. While synthetic oestrogens will usually take care of menopausal hot flushes, they are not without side effects themselves, including vaginal yeast infections, breast tenderness or enlargement, nausea, cramping, bloating, headache/migraine, changes in weight, depression and mood changes. Indeed, it is reported that of the women who choose HRT one-third stop within nine months and more than half within a year due to side effects.

Most healthcare professionals prescribe oestrogen therapy to offset any risk of osteoporosis or heart disease. Unfortunately, studies indicate that as soon as oestrogen therapy is stopped, bone loss escalates, which means a woman would have to remain on the oestrogen forever. Oestrogen's cardiovascular benefits are debatable. Natural health experts agree that there are more appropriate ways to prevent heart disease than by taking prescription oestrogen.

Phytogen is a unique combination of phyto-oestrogens and vitamin E. Herbs containing phyto-oestrogen offer significant advantages over the use of oestrogens in the treatment of menopausal symptoms. While both synthetic and natural oestrogens may pose significant health risks, including increasing the risk of cancer, gall bladder disease and thromboembolic disease (strokes, heart attacks, etc.), phyto-oestrogens have not been associated with these side effects.

Phyto-oestrogens are capable of exerting oestrogenic effects, although the activity is only 2 per cent as strong as oestrogen at the very most. However, because of this low activity, phyto-oestrogens exert a balancing action on oestrogen effects: if oestrogen levels are low, phyto-oestrogens enhance the oestrogen effects; if oestrogen levels are high, phyto-oestrogens reduce the oestrogen effects.

Ingredients

The important compounds contained in *Phytogen* include: soy extract, known to contain saponins which exert an oestrogenic effect; vitamin E, an essential nutrient for cardiovascular function; linseed (flaxseed) oil, rich in lignins, which support hormone function; Gamma-Oryzanol, from rice bran, studied for its relationship to cholesterol levels; and pumpkin seed oil, high in essential fatty acids and sterols.

Each capsule contains:
Vitamin E (D-alpha Tocopherol) 50 iu
Linseed oil 300 mg
Gamma-Oryzanol 100 mg
Pumpkin seed oil (*Curcubita pepo*) 50 mg
Soy extract (non-GMO, standardised to contain 10 per cent
   isoflavones in the forms genistein and diadzin) 20 mg

Capsules also contain glycerin, modified starch, carrageenan,
   disodium phosphate, red iron oxide paste, black oxide paste.
   Excipients: soya bean oil, lecithin, vegetable oil and beeswax.
Contains no gelatin, sugar, salt, yeast, wheat, gluten, corn, dairy,
   artificial flavourings or preservatives.

Dosage
One to three capsules daily as an addition to the everyday diet. *Phytogen* could be taken alongside *Daily Choice for Senior Women*, *Ostivone* or *Osteoprime Forte* for greater support.

Restrictions
None known at stated dosage.

DIINDOLYLMETHANE
Some later findings, like *diindolylmethane*, ensure a very healthy oestrogen metabolism.

What do perimenopause, premenstrual syndrome, enlarged prostate glands and early heart attacks have in common? Oestrogen. A new understanding of healthy oestrogen metabolism is providing a nutritional approach to these and other important health issues confronting both women and men. Fortunately, phytonutrients discovered in cruciferous vegetables offer a natural approach to resolving oestrogen imbalance. Dietary supplementation with an absorbable form of one of these phytonutrients, called *diindolylmethane*, helps promote healthier oestrogen metabolism. Its hormonal balancing effects have revealed that these midlife problems are not due to oestrogen itself, but rather to oestrogen metabolism imbalances.

What is diindolylmethane *and how can it help hormones?*

Diindolylmethane is a phytonutrient (plant nutrient) found only in cruciferous vegetables. These include cabbage, broccoli, Brussels sprouts, cauliflower, kale, kohlrabi, mustard, pak choi, swede and turnip. These plants have been cultivated for thousands of years and were initially used for their medicinal benefits. The connection between *diindolylmethane* and hormones like oestrogen has to do with similar characteristics at the molecular level. It is not an oestrogen or a hormone but, like oestrogen, it shares the common characteristic of being poorly soluble in water. Like oestrogen, it can be metabolised only by a special class of cytochrome enzymes that reside in cell membranes in the non-water part of cells. It turns out that when it is consumed in food or in absorbable formulations, it encourages its own metabolism. This special metabolic pathway for *diindolylmethane*, and the enzymes involved, precisely overlap with the pathway needed for healthy oestrogen metabolism. Stated simply, supplementing the diet with *diindolylmethane* specifically promotes beneficial oestrogen metabolism and helps restore a healthy hormonal balance.

What is oestrogen dominance?

Middle-aged women experience changes in hormone production and metabolism resulting in excess oestrogen action. There are two basic forms of this common imbalance, known as oestrogen dominance.

Perimenopause. In women, slower hormone metabolism in midlife can mean higher-than-normal levels of oestrogen and a deficiency in its healthy metabolites. Faltering oestrogen metabolism often occurs in women during perimenopause (the years before menopause) and is characterised by higher monthly oestrogen levels prior to oestrogen's dramatic fall at menopause. Additionally, progesterone levels fall during perimenopause, resulting in a rising oestrogen-to-progesterone ratio.

Acquired oestrogen imbalance. This important form of oestrogen dominance has to do with inherited problems in oestrogen metabolism and the influence of diet and chemicals on beneficial metabolite production. Acquired oestrogen imbalance affects both men and women.

What benefit can diindolylmethane *offer?*
Supplementing our diets with *diindolylmethane* can shift the production of oestrogen metabolites away from dangerous 16-hydroxy in favour of beneficial 2-hydroxy metabolites. Taking it in an absorbable formulation encourages active and healthy oestrogen metabolism. *Diindolylmethane* supports oestrogen balance by increasing beneficial 2-hydroxy oestrogens and reducing the unwanted 16-hydroxy variety. This improves oestrogen metabolism and helps resolve all three forms of oestrogen dominance.

Why not just eat more cruciferous vegetables?
Recent reports indicate that a higher intake of cruciferous vegetables is associated with a lower risk of prostate cancer. Cruciferous vegetables are protective against hormone-sensitive cancers. However, direct measurements of upward, beneficial shifts in oestrogen metabolism suggest you would have to eat at least two pounds per day of raw or lightly cooked cruciferous vegetables to derive the same benefit as two capsules of specially formulated *diindolylmethane.* Benefits for cervical dysplasia, PMS, BPH (benign prostatic hypertrophy) and other conditions have not been seen with the use of broccoli, cabbage juice, or dried powders or extracts from vegetables. Absorbable *diindolylmethane* formulations overcome the need for active enzymes within the vegetable and chemical reactions in your stomach to produce *diindolylmethane.* For similar reasons, its absorbable formulation provides many advantages over indole-3-carbinol (I3C), another cruciferous phytochemical available as a supplement. I3C is an unstable

precursor that requires activation in the stomach to be converted into *diindolylmethane*. This means I3C must be taken at a much higher dose and can undergo unpredictable and undesirable chemical reactions in your stomach and colon. *Diindolylmethane*, in a delivery system to ensure absorption, is by far preferable to the supplemental use of I3C.

What is the preferred form of diindolylmethane, *according to research?*

Plain *diindolylmethane* is not absorbed due to its poor solubility. When taken as a supplement in a bioavailable formulation, it is well absorbed due to a unique delivery system. In this delivery system, it is absorbed at three times the amount you might derive from two pounds of vegetables. Its use in animals has been associated with preventative benefits for breast and cervical cancer. In humans, supplementation with cruciferous phytonutrients promotes breast, uterine and cervical health. In a study of cervical dysplasia, a recent report documented the disappearance of early cervical cancer over 12 weeks in a placebo-controlled clinical trial.

Supplemental use of absorbable *diindolylmethane* in perimenopausal women has been observed to benefit recurrent premenstrual breast pain and to ease painful menstruation. Its use has been associated with easier weight loss. A number of beneficial activities are attributed to 2-hydroxy oestrogen metabolites, including support for a more active fat metabolism and activity as antioxidants.

How much diindolylmethane *is recommended?*

To replace the *diindolylmethane* from healthy amounts of cruciferous vegetables in the diet, women should take a starting dose of about 15 mg per day of actual *diindolylmethane* in an absorbable formulation. These amounts can be increased three to four times on an individual basis to derive needed benefits for hormonal balance and metabolism.

Since pure *diindolylmethane* must be provided in an absorption-enhancing formulation, the dose for *diindolylmethane* sometimes specifies the weight of the absorbable formulation, which is only one-quarter, or 25 per cent, *diindolylmethane*. In the book *All About DIM* by Michael A. Zeligs and A. Scott Connelly, the suggested dose of 100–200 mg per day for women refers to milligrams of such an absorbable formulation. This dose range for hormonal balance corresponds to 25–50 mg per day of actual *diindolylmethane* for women.

What is the excitement regarding diindolylmethane *and premenstrual syndrome (PMS)?*

PMS symptoms of irritability, aggression, tension, depression, mood swings, water retention and breast pain or swelling are frequently seen in perimenopausal women. While a reduction in PMS severity has been seen with nutritional therapy, full resolution has been elusive. These interventions have included lower fat diets and supplementation with minerals, vitamin D and herbal extracts.

PMS symptom improvement has been noted after beginning dietary supplementation with absorbable *diindolylmethane*. These results suggest it is able to correct the oestrogen imbalance in PMS. Torbjorn Backstrom, MD, an eminent researcher in the field, and others have documented that estradiol, the primary active form of oestrogen, is elevated in PMS. Backstrom has also shown that the degree of estradiol elevation correlates with symptom severity. Also encouraging is the observation that the enzyme pathways promoted by *diindolylmethane* help metabolise pregnenolone sulfate. Pregnenolone sulfate is a brain hormone important for memory, but which causes anxiety if levels are too high. Like oestrogen, pregnenolone sulfate is elevated in PMS. Its healthy metabolism produces beneficial, immune-stimulating metabolites and may help relieve anxiety. Absorbable *diindolylmethane* supplementation promotes healthier metabolism of both oestrogen and pregnenolone in PMS.

What's the best supplemental approach to PMS?

A strong nutritional approach to PMS includes bioavailable *diindolylmethane, chaste berry* extract, vitamin D, calcium and magnesium. Synergistic interaction of these ingredients benefits

PMS in accordance with its physiologic origins. An example of this synergy is the ability for beneficial 2-hydroxy oestrogens to increase progesterone production potentiating this effect by *chaste berry* extract. This new nutritional approach to PMS helps with mineral and hormonal balance. *Diindolylmethane* works in conjunction with *chaste berry* extract to resolve the dominance of oestrogen over progesterone.

Can diindolylmethane *help improve the safety of hormone replacement therapy (HRT)?*
Despite a growing list of benefits attributed to oestrogen, which include younger-looking skin, stronger bones, more comfortable sex and better memory, women often view its potential side effects as unacceptable. A study of postmenopausal women receiving long-term HRT with oestrogen and oestrogen-progesterone combinations has revealed an unequivocal increase in breast cancer risk. Added concerns relate to the increase in the incidence of uterine cancer and an increased risk of life-threatening blood clots, especially after bone fracture. Most recently, the nationwide HERS (Heart and Oestrogen/Progesterone Replacement) study reported the worrying discovery that women with a history of heart disease had an increased risk of heart attack in the first year after starting oestrogen replacement therapy.

Many of oestrogen's risks can be related to a lack of its beneficial metabolites. It is now known that a lower risk of future breast cancer is associated with higher 2-hydroxy oestrogen levels. Supplementation with bioavailable *diindolylmethane* increases protective 2-hydroxy oestrogen and therefore may reduce the risk of HRT-related cancer. Reduction in the risk of abnormal blood clot formation related to HRT oestrogen would benefit women who suffer fractures while on HRT but may also benefit women with early heart disease. It has been known since the Framingham study in Massachusetts that men with the highest estradiol level had the highest risk of early heart attack. *Diindolylmethane* may help normalise the cardiac risk related to unhealthy or underactive oestrogen metabolism in both men and women. Also, the beneficial 2-hydroxy metabolites have been shown to be powerful antioxidants, which may contribute to protecting against the early signs of atherosclerosis and subsequent heart attacks.

Conclusion

Diindolylmethane supplementation is a nutritional approach to achieving a safer and healthier oestrogen metabolism. Many of the benefits traditionally ascribed to oestrogen (protection from heart disease, healthy skin, bones and brain) may actually reside with its beneficial metabolites, the 2-hydroxy oestrogens. *Diindolylmethane* supplementation is a natural promoter of this specific pathway of healthy oestrogen metabolism.

Chapter Four

Cancer of the Cervix

A young, pretty woman called Jennifer once consulted me. She was very businesslike but I could see she was extremely distraught. She told me a little bit about her life, of how she had always been keen to succeed, but her parents had hindered her. Her father was very domineering and her mother was a schoolmistress. She was often prevented from going out when she wanted to and, after leaving school, she tried with difficulty to leave home. When she became a bit older and finally managed to leave, she was unfortunately introduced to drugs and alcohol by friends and also started to believe in free love. This was her biggest downfall, as she told me that she had slept with several boys (and later, men) and had suddenly become very unwell. She was a vegetarian and ate healthily, but nothing seemed to help her. She was bitter about one man in particular, who had slept with her even though he knew he had a sexually transmitted disease. Although Jennifer had only slept with this man a few times, some months later she became ill. After she had a cervical smear test, cancer of the cervix was detected. Luckily, she caught it in time. Treatment of cervical cancer can be very successful if it is detected early.

She asked me to treat her further using natural methods, so I gave her several remedies, but first of all I helped her detox by taking antioxidant remedies. I told her that a great friend of mine, the well-known herbalist Kitty Campion, devised a very good system which I frequently use for people who need enemas to detoxify, and I also advised her to carry out this treatment. Jennifer did very well on the strict diet I advised, carried out the enemas I recommended and also took the prescribed remedies. She could not believe that the man she had slept with had infected her, increasing her risk of developing cervical cancer and, as a result of this, she hated men for a long time. However, she is now full of life and has a partner who makes her happy.

I am often asked about cervical cancer. The cervix is the lower part of the womb. Cancer of the cervix is one of the cancers which occur in the female reproductive system. Others include cancer of the ovaries, the lining of the womb, the vulva and the opening from the vagina. These are mostly termed 'gynaecological cancers'. A lot of women increase their risk of developing cervical cancer by having sex with many different partners. In England and Wales, it is said that about 4,000 women will develop the condition each year. Cervical screening for this problem is excellent in this country. It is therefore essential that a smear test is carried out periodically so that any changes can be detected before cancer has the chance to develop. It only takes a few minutes, but it should definitely be a priority so that action can be taken if necessary. A cervical smear test is a simple procedure and your doctor will be very sympathetic if you are anxious about having it carried out.

Cervical cancer is extremely rare in virgins and the highest risk is to women over 35 years of age. While women are able to examine their breasts, they cannot see or feel the cervix. A smear test is therefore the only way to pick up any problem. Although most results are negative, it is something I often advise patients to do. Any abnormal symptoms should be investigated. The most common symptom of cervical cancer is abnormal bleeding – such as between periods or after intercourse. In women who have been through the menopause (and therefore have stopped their periods) there may be some new bleeding. Of course, there are many other conditions that can produce these symptoms, so it is important to have a smear test carried out to eliminate cancer. Also, when stopping HRT, it is important that an investigation is carried out if there is unexpected bleeding to rule out anything serious. The importance of having smear tests is very well publicised by the Department of Health.

If abnormal cells of the cervix are noticed, the patient is usually advised to have several regular smear tests. Abnormal cells, which are not cancerous but may lead to cancer over a number of years if left untreated, are known as CIN (cervical intra-epithelial neoplasia). There are three different types of CIN – CIN 1, CIN 2 and CIN 3. The treatment is very effective and can be undertaken at an outpatient clinic.

The womb is made up of two parts – the cervix, which is the neck of the womb at the top of the vagina, and the body of the womb which lies in the pelvis above the cervix. There are two main types of cancer of the cervix. The most common form usually develops in the cells which cover the outer surface of the cervix at the top of the vagina and is called squamous cell carcinoma; cancer of the body of the womb develops in the cells which line the cervical canal and is called adenocarcinoma. Although there is no evidence that HRT can increase the chances of developing squamous cell carcinomas, there is always a risk. It becomes much more complicated when endometrial cancer is present, as this has sometimes been linked to HRT dependence. Whilst cancer of the womb can be stimulated by oestrogen or even oestrogen supplements, the use of progesterone does not absolutely guarantee that this disease will not develop.

Due to early detection, the rates of many cervical cancers have luckily been reduced. About 60 years ago, an American doctor called George Papanicolaou devised a test called the Pap smear. This simple method has enabled the early detection of innumerable cervical cancers. The test allows the detection of both early and progressed cervical cancer. It is very simply carried out and involves no pain or discomfort. Pap smear tests should be carried out every three years on healthy women.

Nobody can say what causes cervical cancer. Nevertheless, it is important to realise that whilst there may be many factors involved, a few things should be taken into consideration. As with Jennifer, we often see that if women have many sexual partners, or start having sex too early, the risk is increased. Women who smoke heavily can triple their risk of developing cervical cancer. Passive smoking may also influence the incidence of cervical cancer. With genital infections caused by the human papilloma virus (HPV), which often causes genital warts, cancer of the cervix might develop. HPV is a nasty virus which can easily be transmitted by sexual intercourse. The cervix is very vulnerable, especially in young women. However, a lot can be done during the early stages when changes in the cells (which may lead to cancer and can occur at any age) are detected. If this is the case, it is advisable to discuss treatment with a specialist. The test can be carried out at family planning clinics, well woman clinics or other specialist clinics, as well as at GPs. It will usually take between three to five weeks before the results are known.

It is important to look at effective methods of contraception, which help one to avoid these risks. Non-toxic spermicides and condoms are especially good. I also feel very strongly about the importance of genitourinary medicine clinics, outpatient clinics one can attend if there is any anxiety about possible infection. If you experience any discomfort, such as spots, itching, ulcers or unusual discharge from the vagina, then it is tremendously helpful to visit one of these clinics and allay any fears. If a problem does exist, the doctors there will be able to advise on the appropriate action to take.

I find *Petasan* and *IP-6* very effective remedies for the treatment of cervical cancer.

PETASAN

This remedy contains the herbs butterbur (*Petasites*) and mistletoe (*Viscum album*).

Butterbur has achieved wide recognition as a powerful remedy. Its anti-spasmodic effect eases tension in the cells and reduces susceptibility to pain. It has also been shown to have anti-carcinogenic properties. Some cases have been reported where this simple plant, in conjunction with a change in the patient's lifestyle, has produced remarkable results.

Mistletoe, a peculiar parasitical plant, lives on certain trees. It too has been proven to stimulate the cell metabolism. As this is generally very weak in cancer patients, mistletoe preparations are beneficial for treating the disease. Mistletoe can be given in the form of drops or, in some cases, by injection.

Dosage
Ten drops in half a cup of water, twice a day, after meals.

IP-6 (INOSITOL HEXAPHOSPHATE)
Worldwide, rates of cancer are increasing fast, with over ten million new cases each year. In the UK, cancer is now the single largest killer disease. Statistics like these are alarming, as we tend to think of cancer as being largely unavoidable. It is well known that lung cancer is mainly caused by cigarette smoking and that exposure to sunlight can increase our chances of skin cancer. However, what about other types of cancer whose triggers are less obvious and often multiple in number?

Many of us mistakenly believe that cancer strikes randomly and is unpreventable. In fact, as many as 60–70 per cent of all cancers can be prevented by a healthy diet, an active lifestyle and appropriate use of supplements. In 1997, the World Cancer Research Fund reviewed over 4,000 recent scientific papers and concluded that to avoid cancer our diets should be predominantly plant-based, including at least five portions of fruit and vegetables daily, together with pulses (beans and lentils) and wholegrain cereals. We should limit our intake of red meat, alcohol, salt and processed convenience foods, and avoid tobacco.

Physical activity seems to protect against cancer in general, possibly by maintaining a high proportion of lean tissue to body fat. Exercise is particularly beneficial in protecting against colon cancer – the second most common cancer in women in the UK. It may also reduce the risk of lung cancer and breast cancer – the most common cancers in the UK.

There are many vitamins, minerals and other supplements which may help prevent cancer, either on their own or in combination. One such supplement whose efficacy in preventing cancer and boosting immune function has been demonstrated is IP-6 combined with inositol.

IP-6, otherwise known as phytic acid, is a component of fibre found in wholegrains and legumes (peas and beans). *Inositol* is part of the B-vitamin group and both *IP-6* and *inositol* are found naturally within our body cells, brain, blood and urine. Over 15 years ago, a pathologist, Professor A. Shamsuddin, began research on *IP-6* and *inositol*. He found that *IP-6* acted as an antioxidant and anticancer agent.

For cancers to form and spread, DNA damage within body cells must occur, resulting in an elevated rate of cell division. *IP-6* acts to neutralise the damaging effects of free radicals on body cells and is rapidly taken up by cancer cells, where it normalises their cell division. So, *IP-6* plays a role (1) in preventing the formation of cancer and (2) in the 'turning off' of preformed cancer cells. In its natural form, *IP-6* is poorly absorbed from foods as it forms a complex with protein and various minerals. However, in its purified form, *IP-6* is significantly more bioavailable than that present in wholegrains and legumes.

Inositol is essential for many body functions, including those of the brain, nervous system and reproductive organs. *Inositol* also plays a role in controlling the number and growth of cells. Cancer cells arise in our body on a daily basis and it is the action of *inositol* and related molecules which prevent these cancer cells from multiplying. The addition of *inositol* to *IP-6* was found to enhance the anticancer effect of *IP-6*.

Some of the Science Behind IP-6

- Decreases proliferation of cancerous cells
- Protects against cancer
- Antioxidant
- Enhances activity of natural killer (NK) cells

Inositol, the backbone structure of *IP-6*, has six carbon atoms which have an affinity for phosphate molecules. When all six carbons are bound to phosphate groups, *IP-6* is formed. When only three of the carbons are bound to phosphate molecules, it is called *IP-3*. Professor Shamsuddin discovered that when properly combined with *inositol*, *IP-6* forms two molecules of *IP-3* in the body.

IP-3 plays an important role inside our body cells in cellular communication and the 'turning off' of human cancers, according to *in vitro* studies. Supplementation with *IP-6* plus *inositol* is thought to cause tumour suppression by increasing the concentration of *IP-3*. When levels of *IP-3* in the body are low, cancer cells are able to grow and multiply out of control. However, optimal levels of *IP-3* can significantly reduce cancer cell replication by preventing the manufacture of new DNA. *IP-6* plus *inositol* does not exert the same inhibitory effect in normal, healthy cells. For this reason, it has an important advantage over conventional anticancer agents, such as chemotherapy drugs, which work by killing both cancerous and normal, healthy cells indiscriminately.

An animal study illustrating the efficacy of *IP-6* plus *inositol* involved mice which were administered a compound (DMH) to induce colon cancer formation. One group was given *IP-6* in addition to DMH; another group was given DMH plus *inositol*; a further group was given DMH, *IP-6* and *inositol*. There was also a control group, used to provide a contrast to the experimental groups. The results clearly indicate that the mice treated with either *IP-6* alone or *inositol* alone had reduced occurrence of tumours per animal. This benefit was significantly greater when *IP-6* and *inositol* were given in combination.

	TUMOUR PREVALENCE (per cent mice with tumours)	TUMOUR FREQUENCY (per cent tumours per mouse)
DMH	63	116
DMH + IP-6	47	62
DMH + Inositol	30	45
DMH + IP-6 + Inositol	25	25
Control	0	0

Professor Shamsuddin discovered the proper ratio of *IP-6* and *inositol* to ensure the formation of *IP-3* within the human body and he has witnessed the inhibitory effects of *IP-6* plus *inositol* across wide-ranging cancers including brain, colon, breast, prostate, skin, lung, leukaemia and lymphoma.

It has been found that *IP-6* in combination with *inositol* has the ability to shrink existing cancers *in vitro* and in animal models, but its main use could be in cancer prevention. *IP-6* is also an effective antioxidant. It acts to neutralise the damaging effects of free radicals on body cells and has been shown to enhance immunity by boosting the activity of NK cells. These immune cells protect us by binding to viruses, bacteria and cancer cells and delivering a range of cytotoxic chemicals which effectively destroy these foreign invaders.

IP-6 plus *inositol* has undergone extensive animal testing and human studies. No side effects have been found, either when *IP-6* and *inositol* are used on their own or in combination with conventional chemotherapeutic agents. Indeed, Dr Shamsuddin states that *IP-6* and *inositol* can actually potentiate these treatments.

IP-6 and *inositol* have been found to offer other benefits besides those related to the prevention/treatment of cancer. They also play roles in lowering serum total cholesterol levels, reducing the risk of kidney stones, protecting the heart muscle from damage during a heart attack and preventing complications of diabetes.

IP-6 and *inositol* are found naturally within every body cell. In experimental studies, no adverse side effects have been noted, even with prolonged use at high doses and there are no known drug-nutrient interactions. *IP-6* and *inositol* are available at the Jan de Vries clinics.

The dosage varies depending on individual circumstances. As a general rule, however, healthy people should take two to four capsules daily, between meals; those at special risk of developing disease should take four to eight capsules daily, between meals; and those with active disease should take ten to sixteen capsules (or two scoops of powder) daily, between meals or half an hour before food.

ENEMAS
I find the use of enemas to be particularly important in treating cancer. An enema is also invaluable whenever signs of impending colds, 'flu or digestive problems appear. Although the word 'enema' might invoke feelings of revulsion or embarrassment, they are in fact a very useful aid in the natural healing process. Iridology clearly shows the relation of the colon to all sorts of reflex disease, because the colon is intimately linked to the lymphatic system, the circulation and the nerves by specific reflexes. If any area of the colon is toxic, spastic or inflamed, the symptoms are present not just in the bowel itself but also in the reflex area.

Often when I ask a patient if they are constipated, they unhesitatingly say 'no'. When I question them more closely, it becomes apparent that they believe anything varying from one motion a day to one a week is normal. But surely if you stop and consider it, it is reasonable to suppose that if you eat three times a day, you should be eliminating your intake three times a day. After all, children with good diets and relaxed, healthy systems usually manage about three movements a day without difficulty. If you let food sit in the bowels for three days or, even worse, a week, it deteriorates and putrefies, causing gas, pressure and eventually swellings and pockets which hold further deposits of toxic waste. The poisons from these toxic wastes are then carried throughout the body, causing toxaemia. It is a very rare patient who does not need a good bowel cleanse, followed by a regular maintenance programme to ensure clean, normal, healthy activity of the bowel.

Complete bowel cleansing and maintenance requires specific herbs and diet, both of which will be individually prescribed for you by a health practitioner. Massage helps, as do poultices and packs, and enemas are an indispensable aid to your whole programme.

How to Give Yourself an Enema
First of all, you will need an enema bag, which is available from chemists.

Find a relaxed half hour and something to do while you're retaining the enema (e.g. reading or listening to music). You can take your enema while lying in a warm bath or while lying on a rug on the floor, so that you can go up into the yoga shoulder stand or the posture of the plough, or use a slant board allowing gravity to aid retention. Find out which position you like best.

Fill the enema bag with the douche specifically suggested for your needs (see below), then lie on your back or right side and press the lubricated tip of the enema tube into the rectum until it is firmly in place, using a little oil, Vaseline or KY jelly for lubrication. Release the tube lock or press the plastic enema bag (depending on the type you're using) in a slow, steady motion and let the liquid flow gently into the rectum. Have the liquid at room temperature – too hot and it is uncomfortable, too cold and it is difficult to retain. If the liquid hits a block of impacted faeces, stop the flow, massage the area, turn on to your other side or go up into a shoulder stand. Do one of these things until you're able to inject more liquid. Ideally, you should be able to inject and retain a complete quart of enema fluid for a minimum of ten minutes. If the urge to release simply can't be ignored, it is best to let it go and begin all over again. But you'll find that as the bowel condition improves, it will be easier and easier to accept and retain all the liquid with a minimum of discomfort.

Because the aim is to get the liquid to flow up the descending colon across the transverse and down the ascending colon, it is helpful to change positions and massage the area. Often when a strong urge to release comes, it lasts only for a minute or two and if you breathe quickly and turn your feet at the ankles in a circular motion in both directions, you can ride the storm and you'll find the crisis will pass. Always remember, the greater your need to cleanse using an enema, the more your bowel tries to reject the liquid prematurely. Each time you do an enema, try to hold it a little longer than you did before. Remain lying on the right side or in the inverted posture.

A word of caution: don't overuse enemas, which may result in weakening of the bowel tone. Use them only as part of a complete purification programme and only for as long as instructed.

CANCER OF THE CERVIX

Herbal Enemas

Make a strong infusion of herbal teas or a decoction of roots and barks, strain and cool. Use two teaspoons of herb per pint of water, four teaspoons per quart. This may be made up in advance, but should be used preferably within 24 hours, though certain herbs keep up to 72 hours. However, once souring or scum appears, throw it away. It should be kept in a glass container in a fridge or cool place. Make herbal infusions or decoctions in stainless steel pots only.

Catnip – mildly nervine, calming, soothing, relaxing. Effectively brings down fevers. Excellent for use with children.

Chamomile – excellent for recuperative periods after illness or a healing crisis.

Detoxifying – make a decoction of *yellow dock* and *burdock* roots, then add *red clover* and *red raspberry* infusions. Stimulates the liver to dump bile, thereby relieving stress and pain in a healing crisis.

Slippery Elm – mucilagenous, soothing, softening and nourishing enema. Excellent if the patient is having trouble eating or retaining food, as the bowel absorbs the nutriment.

Sage – warming, purifying.

Garlic – profoundly purifying, an excellent aid in the treatment of worms. Liquidise four cloves in one pint of warm water and strain.

Astringent – *witch hazel, bayberry* or *white oak bark,* used to help stop diarrhoea and dysentery.

Flaxseed – relieves inflammation, pain and bleeding (more effective if you add two teaspoons of liquid chlorophyll). Also aids the healing process.

Coffee Enemas

The coffee enema is widely publicised these days as a part of cancer therapy and chronic care naturopathy. It is an excellent way to relieve healing crisis pain and discomfort, to stimulate the liver to dump bile by absorption of the coffee into the haemorrhoidal veins and the portal veins, and to encourage deep cleansing of the colon by stimulating peristaltic activity. The coffee enema is prepared by putting three tablespoons of ground coffee beans into one quart of distilled water which has just been brought to the boil. Continue on the boil for three minutes and then simmer on very low heat for 20 minutes. Cool. Strain and inject while at body temperature. Retain for 10–15 minutes.

This can be done every morning when on a detoxification programme or fast, and every hour during an acute healing crisis. The bowels continue to operate independently even when one is using the coffee enema regularly and start functioning easily on their own after the treatment is discontinued. The coffee enema is recommended after a lymph massage, to cleanse the colon of the lymph which has drained into the bowel, but not before sleep, as it is too stimulating. Herbal substitutes for the coffee enema are: *red clover, yellow dock root, burdock* and *red raspberry*.

Spirulina Enema

The use of spirulina plankton enemas, together with fasting and purification programmes, is an excellent way to cleanse the colon and purify the bloodstream as quickly as possible. Spirulina has the unique advantage of supplying strength and power through the absorption of the plankton into the bowel wall, as well as cleansing at the same time by softening the impacted faecal matter and stimulating peristalsis. Direct nutrition absorbed by the colon provides proteins and essential amino acids, laying a balanced foundation for easy purification, since hunger and weakness are prevented by the spirulina intake. The spirulina enema may be made as follows: heat one blender-full of distilled water to body temperature. Mix two teaspoons of spirulina powder with half a cup of cold water till you make a smooth paste. Add two teaspoons of glycerine (available from chemists) and stir together. Add this loose paste to a blender, half full of the warm distilled water, and mix at a slow speed. You can also use a whisk. Add the remaining distilled water slowly to fill the blender. Fill the enema bag right away and use quickly.

This method will wash out the lower and upper bowel and encourage a complete peristaltic downward action. The plankton is also absorbed into the bowel wall, helping to soften, loosen and dilute the bowel contents. Inject the mixture a little at a time while lying on the right side. Move back and forth from the left to the right side, and massage the bowel area. If you feel that retention is impossible, then eject and start the process over again. With practise, the bowel becomes accustomed, and eventually you will be able to retain a full enema of two quarts for five to ten minutes, while massaging the abdomen. Use of the shoulder stand will help the spirulina to reach throughout the intestinal tract. The glycerine helps to emulsify the mixture, soften the impacted faeces and lubricate the walls of the colon. Take the enema the first night of any fast and for the next two nights. While you continue the fast, take one every other day and, after the fast, take once a month on a regular basis for effective bowel maintenance. Spirulina powder is better than grinding tablets, being without additives.

Castor Oil Packs
Castor oil packs assist enemas, because the absorption of the castor oil via the skin into the lymphatic system and lacteals in the small intestines softens, relaxes, nourishes and balances the sympathetic and parasympathetic nervous systems. It also disperses congestion and tension and slowly helps to release any blockages in the bowel pockets. The herbalist Dr Christopher comments, 'Castor oil helps to get rid of hardened mucous in the body, which may appear as cysts, tumours or polyps.'

1. Soak a 100 per cent-cotton flannel in castor oil and place over entire abdomen.
2. Cover with a second moist flannel to provide wet heat.
3. Cover these two layers with plastic.
4. Place a heating pad over the top.

5. Cover everything with a thick towel which wraps around to hold the layers in place.
6. Enjoy this soothing and relaxing pack for one and a half hours, three days in a row.
7. For the next three days, massage the entire area with olive oil.
8. Rest on the seventh day and then repeat.

One of the happy results of a clean colon is a more stable emotional life. It is said among natural healers that the constipated person is an irritable, impatient one. If we could only realise consciously the importance of internal hygiene on our general health, well-being and appearance, we would balance all our efforts for external appearance with internal cleanliness. It is certainly an essential aspect of any body-cleansing programme, whether for preventive or curative treatment. Once it is accepted into your life and has a place as accepted as other beauty and health routines, you will be able to apply it when needed for beneficial results. Many people have a psychological resistance to enemas and it is hoped this information will help you to overcome that. Your life will be the better for this knowledge.

It is necessary to keep a careful eye on any worrying situation so that the increase of cancer may be reduced by the introduction of such methods.

Chapter Five

Ovarian Cancer

Following tests on a large number of symptom-free women, research has shown that ovarian cancer can be detected early. This is known as screening. You will firstly be asked to give a blood sample. There is a substance called CA 125, a protein, that is present in most women's blood. The level may be higher in women with ovarian cancer, as it is sometimes produced by ovarian cancer cells and this can be detected by the test. The problem with the test, however, is that there are too many false negatives to use it as a general screening tool. Many women can have an elevated level of CA 125 but do not have ovarian cancer. Some factors which cause CA 125 levels to be elevated include endometriosis, pelvic inflammatory disease, uterine fibroids, ectopic pregnancy, menstruation, first trimester pregnancy, or heart or renal failure. In the research trials, it was shown that ovarian cancer can be detected at a fairly early stage.

Cancer of the ovaries is one of the cancers that can occur in the female reproductive system. The disease can also be present in the endometrium, the cervix, the entrance of the womb or the vulva. Annually, ovarian cancer affects many women annually and although it is most common in women over the age of 50, it can affect women of any age. However, as women get older, their chance of developing ovarian cancer increases. This is particularly the case after menopause and usually peaks around the ages of 60 to 75. Sometimes ovarian cancer can be linked to a faulty gene, while in other cases it can be a dietary matter. It is very important that any lumps, fibroids (or cysts as they are often called) are examined. Women who have ovarian cancer often overlook symptoms because they are mild and not very noticeable. These may include indigestion, a bloated feeling, unexplained weight gain, pain in the lower abdomen, loss of appetite, vaginal bleeding, or changes in bowel and bladder habits – all small indications that may pinpoint ovarian cancer.

This type of cancer can also run in families. The genes related to ovarian cancer are tumour suppressor genes: they normally prevent or suppress a cell growth. Quite a number of women who carry faulty inherited genes are at risk of developing ovarian cancer. One often reads of HNPCC, which stands for hereditary non-polyposis colorectal cancer. This is often a development of cancer of the bowel or cancer of the ovaries. In a large number of cases, this abnormal gene can be identified in women who have it in their families.

British researchers have discovered a gene that can stop ovarian cancer from developing, which is a significant advance in the understanding of the disease known as 'the silent killer'. Each year 2,600 women are diagnosed with ovarian cancer. Nearly 1,500 of them die. This is an extremely high percentage and clearly indicates that the present treatment offered to ovarian cancer patients is not as successful as it should be. Researchers have found a gene called OPCML, which was tested on fully established ovarian tumours and seemed to dramatically suppress their growth. This dramatic breakthrough represents an exciting advance in ovarian cancer research and could aid researchers in finding a method of earlier diagnosis and treatment of this disease.

I clearly remember a lady who had flown from Cornwall and was brought to me on a stretcher for her first consultation. She had inoperable, widespread ovarian cancer and had a letter from her doctor stating that she had only a month to live. Twenty-eight years later, I met her on the stair of my clinic in Harley Street – singing. When I commented that she seemed rather happy, she replied, 'I have every reason to be. You cured me 28 years ago.' I told her I do not cure anyone – God cures, I only treat, and she had done a lot to help herself. She had been on very strong hormonal treatments which offered her no relief until she finally gave up and decided that she had to change her lifestyle completely. She hated the small glasses of beetroot juice I used to give her each morning and, basically, detested everything about the diet I prescribed for her, which consisted mainly of fruit and vegetables with no meat at all. I do not always forbid meat, but in her case it was necessary. She loved eating meat and, as a tremendous amount of meat contains hormones, I felt that this might have been the trigger to her developing cancer. This lady had survived on a poor diet, but she had forgotten to ask herself the big questions, 'Are these hormones safe? Is there a "risk-to-benefit" factor? Is there a "no risk" factor through diet and nutrition?'

Hormones naturally originate from internal secretions of the 'ductless' glands (pituitary body attached to the brain, thyroid and parathyroid in the neck, the pancreas, the islets of Langerhans, adrenals, near the kidneys, and gonads in the scrotum or pelvic cavity). These glands produce an internal secretion which is discharged into the blood or lymph and circulated to all parts of the body. Hormones, the active principles of the glands, produce effects more or less remote from their place of origin. As scientists learned more about the vital functions, actions and reactions resulting from glandular secretions, it became popular to experiment with administering firstly animal secretions and then synthetic drugs to humans. Both methods produced results – some were beneficial and others caused adverse reactions. In a few unfortunate cases, it became apparent that a small percentage of recipients of glandular therapy (mostly women) developed cancer and the 'risk-to-benefit' factor was given serious consideration.

Since hormones are necessary to life in animals and human beings, nature must have originally had a built-in plan for the generation and regeneration of hormone production within the body itself. Further research has revealed that plants also make hormones. Among them are the auxins, rich and vigorous in the sprouts of seeds (especially at the early stage of the sprouting process). Research concerning auxins of oat sprouts and castrated roosters proved the value of hormone precursors – the nutrients from which the body can 'manufacture' hormones. The castrated roosters regained some of their male characteristics, developing new red combs and pursuing the hens. Today, it has been found that other hormone precursors include the nuclei of various seeds, a highly concentrated source of germ oil fractions. These hormone precursor nutrients are suitable for those to whom hormone medication may pose an unnecessary risk. Adding whole, unrefined grains, wheat germ and sprouts to the daily diet can provide real benefits.

We must not forget that almost half of all men and women in the United States will be diagnosed with cancer or cancerous growths. Cancer develops when cells are out of control as a result of damage to DNA in their nuclei. Cancers will attract new blood vessels to themselves to feed their runaway appetite for the nutrients they require. They can even clone themselves and travel through the bloodstream into the lymphatic system. Certain foods can negatively produce cancer cells which use energy at a rate of up to 70 times that of a healthy cell. The war is on and to prevent and control this terrific growth, a wholesome diet and various remedies are necessary.

Cancer is a devastating disease. There can be so many causes of it: genetic predisposition and mutations, and abnormalities in the nuclei of the cell caused by chemicals, radiation, hormones and viruses, accounting for 5–10 per cent and 90–95 per cent of all cancers respectively. There are many different approaches to the treatment of cancer, but as a cancer cell grows so rapidly, often chemotherapy or radiotherapy is necessary to halt its growth. One should, however, never forget that in this warfare it is necessary to build a healthy cell to replace each cancerous one that is destroyed by the treatment. A tumour cell grows and replicates much more rapidly than a normal cell because they are better equipped to receive glucose, having seven times more insulin receptors and ten times more ITF receptors than normal cells. Also, cancer cells quickly develop a network of blood vessels (angiogenesis) to ensure an efficient supply of nutrients and oxygen. Ongoing studies have shown that much of this process can be stopped with the use of safe remedies, as well as the adoption of a wholesome diet.

It was heart-warming recently when a husband and wife came into my busy surgery. The gentleman showed me a letter from the hospital which said that his wife's cancerous tumour had mysteriously disappeared. He asked me if I knew who his wife was and I told him that I knew her as a patient, but no more than that. He then told me that he and his wife were consultants in a hospital. He was almost certain that the administration of *IP-6* had probably done the trick. I told him that *Petasan* with *IP-6* is an excellent combination of remedies. It is often a very successful treatment for inoperable tumours. His wife was prepared to adopt the correct dietary management, but it took a lot of willpower for her, especially to give up meat from the pig – pork, sausages, bacon, ham and gammon. For her, as with the first lady I mentioned in this chapter, meat, milk and cheese (particularly cow's milk cheese, because of the hormone influence) were forbidden foods. When the meat is not organic, it can be dangerous to our health. Dietary management is extremely important, as is looking after the immune system. As I have so often said in lectures, one cannot reach this goal by eating a synthetic pudding or a tin of tomato soup that has never seen a real tomato!

MEAT
In the past, meat was quite different to what it is now. Then, a healthy animal which grazed on unpolluted grass provided much healthier meat than that which is available today.

For a long time, meat was a luxury most people could not afford. Later on, it gradually became cheaper and now almost everyone can afford it. Today, meat has been given the place of honour, while vegetables and other healthy foods do not seem to be very important to most people who live in the industrial countries.

Do We Need Meat?
There are millions of people in the world who do not eat meat and are nevertheless healthy. What we eat is very personal and our choice

to eat meat or abstain from it is no different. Although the meat we eat today is certainly not one of our healthiest foods, there are people who obviously need the satisfaction which they derive from its inclusion in their diet. It seems to give them a pleasure that one could call addictive. If such people do not eat meat more than twice a week, it will probably not harm them; the pleasure they find in eating will counterbalance the possible negative effects meat may have on their health. Here 'mind over matter' is very important.

Many religions do not permit the consumption of pork. This is not only for religious reasons. Pork meat contains fat which provides an ideal living condition for germs and viruses and can therefore cause all kinds of diseases. For this reason, pork is definitely not a healthy food.

Eating Meat Can Cause Illness

Since meat has become cheaper, its consumption has increased phenomenally. There are people who eat up to 80 kilograms or even more meat per year. The human organism does not have the ability to process such vast amounts of meat.

As soon as an animal has been killed, the meat starts to decompose and because of this, meat eaters always get a leucocytosis (an increase in white blood cells) and their stools usually smell foul. Meat eaters often suffer from constipation, as muscle meat lacks fibre (roughage).

With the aid of a capillary microscope, one can see that the capillaries (tiny blood vessels) are often damaged as a consequence of eating meat. During an average lifetime, the net of these tiny blood vessels shrinks from initially 100,000 kilometres to about 50,000. When meat is digested, many toxic acids develop; these put a big strain on the liver and the kidneys. At first, these acids are stored as crystals in the body tissues, but later they enter the cells and cause gout, rheumatism, diabetes, obesity, kidney disease and neuralgia.

Which Meat Does Most Harm?

For a long time, it has been known that pork and everything which is made from it, such as bacon, ham, sausages, etc., is bad for our health and the latest scientific research reveals that poultry and veal are not good for us either. This kind of meat seems to dissolve very quickly in the human body and can, within a short time, inundate the blood with so much acid that even the healthiest body cannot cope with it.

The quality of meat can be very variable. The meat of an animal that has roamed about the Argentinian pampas and eaten food which is 100 per cent natural is certainly much healthier than that of an animal from an industrial country, which receives twice a day its portion of so-called 'power fodder'. Formerly, such special food consisted of cereals and other natural products, like soya beans, which fulfilled the needs of the animals in an optimal way. However, the major part of today's 'power fodder' not only endangers the health of the animals, but could also cause very serious disease in millions of human beings.

Concentrated Fodder and Disease
Could you imagine a lion living on grass and vegetables? Certainly not! Very soon, such a lion would become seriously ill and die. Everybody is able to understand this. A lion is a carnivore, a meat eater, and its digestive organs could never digest different food.

On the other hand, grass and raw vegetables are the right food for cows and other herbivorous animals. A cow is a plant eater and its digestive system, with its three stomachs, is designed exclusively to digest grass and other vegetation. If a cow swallows a few ants or beetles, it will not come to any harm. However, a few decades ago, profit-conscious manufacturers came up with an idea which was not only extremely dangerous, but also quite unbelievable. In order to make more money, they began to treat cows and other plant eaters like carnivorous animals! Cows now eat meat! Many people cannot believe this, but it is the truth. Of their own accord, cows would never even touch meat, but years ago industry got the wonderful idea of using a trick so that cows would not know what they were eating. This same trick has been used to fool people for a long time.

Foul-tasting meat residues and remains are, with flavourings that are exactly adapted to the taste of the animals, changed into real 'gourmet' foods for cows. The very high protein content of this 'power fodder' guarantees that calves will grow quickly, cattle will gain weight and cows will give much more milk (up to 15 litres per day).

The production of this kind of fodder has become big business. Through its use, industry has been able to solve two serious problems. As meat consumption has, during the last 100 years, increased at least five-fold, the disposal of millions of animal carcasses, which in the past was costly and troublesome, is now very profitable. Concentrated food made from soya or cereals was very expensive and had to be imported. Since then, animal waste processing has become a booming business.

Animal Waste Processing Factories (Knackers' Yards)

There are recycling plants throughout the western world where dead animals and meat residues are made into meal for animal fodder. These are horrible places, very dirty and evil-smelling, where fat, blood, intestines, bones, heads, tails as well as entire bodies of cows, pigs, sheep, chickens and other animals are processed. Although the dead animals are checked at random to ascertain if they are healthy, it is quite impossible to detect certain diseases in the initial stages and there always remains a certain risk of infectious diseases.

The Wrong Fuel

No animal can stay healthy when it is forced to eat food it cannot really digest. The same thing happens when the engine of a car gets the wrong type of fuel. Gradually the engine will deteriorate and eventually break down. A young calf which is fed with the above-mentioned fodder will grow faster, but it will never be as healthy as a calf which gets the right fodder. Such an animal loses its natural defences against all kinds of bacteria and infections. On the one hand, these animals get too much protein, on the other hand this alien food lacks many of the essential nutrients cows need in order to be healthy.

Although cows give more milk and cattle put on more muscle meat, they are no longer strong and healthy animals. They are ill more often and need more and more antibiotics and other drugs. Some of these are prohibited and can only be obtained on the black market. Many of them cannot be completely broken down in the body of the animal and when we eat meat or drink milk, a small part of these will be assimilated into our body.

The Danger Increases – BSE

In the beginning, farming was doing well and the animals seemed to be quite healthy. Then, about 25 years ago, more and more cattle started to suffer from BSE, also known as 'mad cow disease'. The scientific name for this disease is bovine spongiform encephalopathy. Before long it came to light that sheep which were infected with this illness had eaten contaminated power fodder. Cattle and other animals, including zoo cats, which had eaten contaminated food became ill and died. More and more veterinarians and scientists became very concerned about what was happening. The animals suffering from this illness showed the typical symptoms of a cerebral disease. They became nervous and vicious, their whole bodies trembled and they were no longer able to coordinate their movements. After a while, they collapsed and died. Soon BSE became a catastrophe which was more and more widespread.

In Britain, a well-known nutrition expert demanded the slaughter of millions of cattle. Actually, only about a quarter of a million were killed, but this almost brought about a crisis in the British Government. In some European countries which had been importing British cattle for many years, the first BSE cases were reported.

BSE is an encephalopathy (a disease of the brain) which can be transferred orally – that is, via food. The BSE epidemic, especially in Britain, had been spreading and, after some years, in 1990, it was realised that there was also an unusual increase of a certain cerebral disease in people. This is called Creutzfeldt-Jakob disease (CJD) and it affects the central nervous system. Although it was officially denied that BSE and CJD had anything to do with each other, it was still very frightening. We know that CJD can take 20 years to develop and although many respected scientists seem to be sure that it is impossible for humans to be infected with BSE, other experts are not convinced of this.

Scientific research revealed that many animals suffering from BSE showed the same symptoms as those found in people who have certain diseases of the brain. Not only in the case of CJD, but also when people have Alzheimer's disease or multiple sclerosis, some parts of the brain show an extensive degeneration of brain cells. Such diseases are not infectious diseases in the usual sense, as there are no normal reactions of the immune system in order to fight the infection. A hereditary disposition has, as far as we know, little to do with them and therefore many scientists agree that these diseases are caused by – up until now – unknown disease-provoking mechanisms.

It is absolutely logical, if they are eating the wrong kind of food, which they cannot digest, that not all animals will be healthy and that they will, after some time, become chronically ill. The meat of weak and diseased animals can never be healthy for us and it is far worse when these animals have been infected by other diseased animals. The big problem is that the incubation period (the time it takes from the earliest beginning until the actual development of a disease) can be very long. Until the disease is diagnosed (and the animal may already have been ill for some time before this happens), it is almost impossible to prevent the transmission of such diseases.

Some years ago, after sensational newspaper reports and programmes referring to this problem, people became very frightened and many no longer wished to eat meat at all. But after a while things got back to normal and now it seems that the danger has passed.

Is there really no more danger? Nobody knows for sure. The authorities certainly took adequate measures to protect the public, but nobody knows exactly what fodder cattle and other slaughter animals are being fed in their home country or abroad. There are still so many unanswered questions. Do they now get the expensive soya or cereal fodder? Are all the animal recycling plants still operating? How many animal waste-processing plants are there in Europe or in other parts of the world? Which imported meat from which countries still comes from healthy animals?

And did cows finally get used to the idea of being treated like carnivorous animals? Of course, they will never get used to it and, in consequence, all these animals will degenerate and, in the long run, become diseased. Although the danger of BSE seems to have passed, there is still a much greater danger – and that is the ignorance and stupidity of people who think they know better than nature.

Many questions are still open – questions which apparently are not important any more. Meanwhile, the increase of brain and nervous diseases has become frightening. Could there be a connection between those diseases and certain eating habits? Why is there hardly any scientific research done in this area? Probably you can guess why!

In the meantime, we continue to eat what we like and many of us still love to consume meat. However, to be on the safe side, it would be advisable to eat a little less of it in future.

WHAT ELSE CAN WE EAT?

After reading this, you will surely ask what kind of food you *can* still eat. It seems that everything we like to eat is forbidden and unhealthy. Mainly for this reason and because there are so many different opinions about what is healthy and unhealthy, most people do not even start to change their eating habits. While one is still young and more or less healthy, this does not seem to be very important. However, by the time one gets older and is no longer as healthy, or even suffering from some chronic disease, things are different.

As more than 70 per cent or, according to some people, more than 90 per cent, of all our civilisation's diseases are caused by modern nutrition, even the best doctor cannot cure such a disease if the patient does not change his or her nutritional habits.

Healthy food can be varied, very tasty and can be adjusted to all personal likes and dislikes. You should not alter your eating habits drastically straight away. Many patients, realising that this is their last chance to get well, change their diet quite suddenly and this is wrong. After a few days, people who do this often get stomach-ache and other complaints and become convinced that this so-called healthy food does not agree with them. They are discouraged and no longer make the effort to eat differently. They go back to eating the same kind of food as before and their disease becomes worse.

If, however, the change of diet has been made gradually, after some weeks or even days there will be a positive change in the state of health. This becomes a real challenge and when symptoms go away, the person in question is delighted.

While changing the diet, the patient's reaction to different kinds of food should always be taken into consideration and the changes should be made step by step. Taking it easy is the best way.

Changing Your Diet

The first thing you should do is eliminate from your menu the foods which do most harm, and these are all denatured industrialised foods. This means that:

1. You should eat less and less refined sugar, flour and fats, or foods containing these products. If this is difficult for you, in the beginning you can use honey, pure maple syrup or something similar. For some people a change of diet will be more difficult than for others, especially for those who were used to eating many sweets and desserts. However, it is interesting that, after a period of eating only natural sweets like honey or sweet fruits, the craving for sugar disappears.

2. Someone who was used to eating big helpings and often eating between meals now has to get used to eating only half the quantity. This is not difficult to learn if you take a smaller portion each time and if you chew each bite for longer. Perhaps in the beginning you will be hungry between meals and perhaps you will get tired more quickly. In that case, you can eat (slowly!) one or two pieces of fruit, or in case this does not help, you can eat a small portion of boiled unsweetened oats instead of fruit.

Of course, in the beginning, you will probably make many mistakes and might be easily tempted to eat something unhealthy.

However, after some time you will get used to the new way of eating. Surprisingly, after a while sweets will not taste as good as they did before and after eating something that is not so healthy, you will not feel as good. Usually there is a great improvement in one's health and one can enjoy life again.

After some weeks, when you have become used to eating healthier food, you can take the next step on the road to health. From now on, eat no more than three times a day at the most, without any snacks – the only exception being some fruits. This allows the digestive system to take a rest in between meals.

For breakfast, eat fruit, a well-prepared muesli or some whole-wheat bread with a little butter and honey, or a hearty spread from the health food shop. With this, you can drink herbal tea or decaffeinated coffee with a little cream, but no sugar.

At midday, start with a little bowl of salad, with the right kind of salad dressing (some cold-pressed oil, a little lemon juice or apple vinegar, some sea salt or herbal salt and herbs). After the salad, you can eat two or three kinds of steamed vegetable, a jacket potato, whole rice, polenta or another cereal dish. Never use any kind of fat or oil during the preparation of these foods. When they are on your plate, you can add a little butter or cold-pressed vegetable oil. You can eat meat, fish or eggs two or three times a week in the beginning, but after that you should eat less of these foods.

With the exception of soy beans or sprouts, I cannot recommend soya or similar products. All processed foods lose much of their original value with each step of the process. Soya and similar foods are intensively processed and they cannot possibly contain many ingredients which are valuable for our health after this process has been completed. Everyone will basically understand this. Wholemeal cereals are far healthier, as the biological origin of new and foreign products is uncertain.

Especially in the beginning, your meals should always be as simple as possible – a vegetable dish, a cereal dish or soup, muesli or something similar. If, at the beginning, you still want to drink coffee or black tea, it does not matter. However, if your disease is serious and you want to get completely well, you should follow all the advice given. Although a change of diet is extremely important, this nutritional therapy should, especially in the case of serious and chronic diseases, be supported by natural healing methods and remedies.

Chapter Six

Uterine Cancers

The most common type of cancer affecting the womb is called endometrial carcinoma, which develops in the cells lining the inside of the womb. Although this cancer is now much less common, there are still a few hundred new cases each year in the UK. There are several types of sarcomas of the uterus:

- Carcinosarcomas: these make up about four out of ten uterine sarcomas and are often called mixed Mullerian tumours or malignant mixed mesodermal tumours
- Leiomyosarcomas: these also account for about four out of ten uterine sarcomas
- Endometrial stromal tumours make up less than two out of ten out of this group
- A mixed group of unclassified and aggressive sarcomatous cancers make up the remainder

There are signs that sarcomas of the womb are becoming more common. Lower abdominal or pelvic pains, or vaginal bleeding are the commonest symptoms. Surgery is often necessary, although the condition might be treated in other ways.

If the lymph nodes are not removed or the tumour looks more aggressive when examined under a microscope after surgery, or if it invades deeply into the muscle wall of the uterus, then radiotherapy is often necessary. If the sarcoma comes back after treatment, additional treatment is called for. The outlook for women with uterine sarcomas is very variable. Sometimes intense treatment is necessary.

Cancer of the womb (endometrial cancer) occurs in the female reproductive system and affects many women worldwide. The bleeding caused by these cancers must be stopped and patients have to follow the strict guidelines given to them. With these particular cancers, *IP-6* is often very helpful, as well as vitamin, mineral and trace element therapy, which should be devised individually for each patient. This also relates to cancer of the vulva. Although it is rare, cancer of the vulva causes a lot of bleeding, itching and burning and can give great discomfort. This cancer can be the result of overuse of HRT. It is always important to follow strictly the regime advised.

Although the causes of some vaginal cancers are unknown, research is continually going on in an attempt to discover more. There are also some very rare types of vaginal cancer. Cases of these diseases are on the increase and it is therefore crucial that the slightest symptoms are investigated as soon as possible. It is a good idea, particularly if blood is noticed when passing urine, that a full pelvic examination is carried out, especially if there is also bleeding after sexual intercourse. Cervical smears or colposcopies provide an accurate picture of any problems and can be undertaken quickly. Biopsies can also show any abnormal areas.

Again we ask ourselves – how and why do these problems occur? Although viruses, infections and parasites play a role, there is still a big question mark over their cause. One thing is for sure, dietary management is necessary during treatment and is often of great help, together with the inclusion of beneficial remedies. It is also important to look at the immune system, which we shall do in the next chapter.

At present mainstream medicine still does not understand that our 'new' diseases have a completely different origin to the formerly more common infectious diseases. It is careless and irresponsible to treat such completely different diseases in exactly the same manner as infections would be treated. As Hippocrates said, 'The first law while treating a patient is never to do any harm.' However, a host of physicians, often without realising it, offend almost daily against this law!

HEALTHY BLOOD

I am often asked whether it is true that cancer is a blood disease. Of course it is important that we have healthy blood. Before nutrients from a healthy, well-balanced diet are absorbed into the blood, they pass through innumerable small filters located in the intestinal wall. Then the nutrients are cleaned and absorbed by the capillaries (the tiniest blood vessels). These countless capillaries, situated directly behind the intestinal wall, then come together in a wide channel, the portal vein (*vena porta*), which leads to the liver. The liver is our most important detoxifying organ. There the blood is again cleaned by innumerable tiny filters before being absorbed into the general bloodstream, together with the oxygen-containing blood from the lungs.

We have, so to speak, two different kinds of blood, the arterial and the venous blood. The arterial blood (which flows from the heart) contains all the nutrients and oxygen needed by our body cells. Its flow is almost as light as water and it has a nice red colour due to its oxygen content. The venous blood (which flows to the heart) provides, in cooperation with the lymphatic fluid, the detoxification and disposal of harmful or useless materials.

Our blood flows through our body in channels which become smaller and smaller. From these capillaries, it finally flows into the tissues, where it comes into contact with the body cells. Here, the so-called 'metabolic exchange' takes place. This means that the cells now choose and absorb from the arterial blood those nutrients which they require for their individual needs. Meanwhile, the venous blood absorbs the waste products of the cells. Only certain specific waste products are transported directly via the lymph tract to the lymphatic glands, where they are detoxified. Then all the different residues are transferred to the excretory organs, where they are disposed of.

If, once in a while, we overeat or indulge ourselves with unhealthy food, this miracle machine can repair the damage and restore health. Nobody has to be a health fanatic. Our body is a living miracle machine. However, it is now known that normal cell metabolism and function depend mainly on the quality of the nutrients which are supplied by the blood.

From a naturopath's point of view, unhealthy blood is blood of inferior quality. The quality of the blood changes when there are fluctuations in the mineral, trace element and vitamin metabolism; when the blood fats are too high or too low; and when the protein values, acid-alkaline metabolism and blood-clotting processes are abnormal. When any of those factors are present there is the possibility of congestion and infection. As a result of the poor quality of most modern food, which can cause obstructions or permeability of the tiny blood filters, many people nowadays have blood that is of an inferior quality.

These small filters are able to filter only a certain amount of blood at one time, and when there are too many noxious substances, a build-up of such substances in the portal vein may develop. An accumulation of harmful substances can, in turn, create an accumulation of blood in the abdomen, and thus be the cause of the development of a so-called 'collateral circulation'. This means that the organism, in order to prevent greater dangers, will create new blood vessels which can divert the superfluous blood. As a consequence, haemorrhoids or varicose veins can develop, as well as the unsightly small veins on the thighs which are always an indication of blood accumulation in the larger blood vessels.

Sometimes insufficiently filtered blood can get directly into the general blood circulation. Such blood contains many irritating substances and the red blood cells in the finest blood vessels mass together, the blood cells become less mobile and the blood circulation is diminished.

When the circulation is diminished, many cells cannot be fed properly. At first, it is mainly the cells in the periphery of the body that do not get enough nutrients and the blood circulation in the feet and often in the hands stagnates. More and more people today complain about cold feet. Before long, more toxic substances are deposited in the tissues. These penetrate deep into the body and all the time damage is being done.

There can also be another reason for poor circulation and that is the intake of too much protein, which the oncologist Professor Wendt has described so well and which causes very high blood pressure. It is bad for the health when too much protein, especially animal protein, is eaten. The human body is not able to use all of it. In such a case, the superfluous protein is deposited in the walls of the capillaries in such a way that they eventually become clogged and the blood can no longer pass. Circulation problems, high blood pressure, hardening of the arteries, early diabetes, rheumatic diseases and gout can occur.

The correct therapy for these diseases would be protein fasting. In any case, the nutrition of the patient should contain very little protein and bloodletting, cupping and other natural healing methods and remedies should be prescribed and carried out by a qualified practitioner.

Let me state that for any diet to be successful, there should be total trust between the patient and the practitioner. In fact, that applies to any treatment therapy. The following advice is also useful:

- To help good digestion, take plenty of rest
- Do not get overtired
- Make sure you take outdoor exercise for good oxygen flow
- Remain optimistic
- Do not hesitate to ask friends and family for their support
- Be positive

Chapter Seven

Cancer and the Immune System

I saw a lady today for the first time in 38 years. I recalled our very first consultation, when she told me that she had stomach cancer and thought she would not survive. Nevertheless, she asked if I would treat her. I informed her that only oncologists are permitted to treat cancer patients in this country, but I would do my best to strengthen her immune system and make her body strong enough to cope with the treatments that lay ahead of her. I explained that there was a war going on in her body and the chemotherapy would not only kill the cancerous cells but also the healthy ones. The best thing I could do for her was to back up the hospital treatment she would be receiving.

She was very happy to cooperate with me and, when I examined her, I could see that her immune system had deteriorated quite considerably. She was also extremely anaemic and had very little reserves with which to fight. I was so worried about her that I phoned one of my best friends that evening. I regard him as one of the best immunologists in this country and I asked him if he knew how the immune system really works. He told me that although he had written many books on this subject, he still did not know for certain.

Today, not only with cancer and leukaemia, but with any disease – particularly infectious disease – it is of great importance that we nurture and care for our immune system. But what is the immune system? The body's defence system includes three main types of immune cell:

- B-lymphocytes
- T-lymphocytes
- macrophages (scavenger cells)

B-lymphocyte cells are made from bone marrow and are responsible for the production of antibodies. However, all three types of immune cells found in the body work together in attacking bacteria, foreign invaders and toxic substances such as cancer and viruses.

In order for the immune system to develop properly and be able to combat cancer cells, not only natural proteins are needed, but also the essential amino acids – for adults and children alike. Also necessary are vitamins A, B5, B6, B12 and C, iron, folic acid, biotin, selenium, zinc, pantothenic acid, magnesium, copper and essential fatty acids such as GLA (gamma linolenic acid) or oil of evening primrose. All these substances are capable of boosting the immune system.

Vitamin A helps to regulate the system and a lack of it will cause a deficiency in T-lymphocyte cells. The B vitamins will help to increase the production of thymus hormones. Linolenic acid is needed to support the essential fatty acids. Evening primrose oil, together with linolenic acid, will help the levels of prostaglandins, which also help the T-lymphocyte cells in the immune system.

In the thymus glands of young animals, substances are formed that have the ability to transform lymphocytes. So-called T-lymphocytes recognise the bacteria and viruses that have invaded the cells and attack them. Alien albumen and degenerated cells are likewise rendered innocuous through this defence mechanism. In the human organism, after puberty the thymus gland gradually reduces the level of production of these substances which are so important for defence. By the age of 40, the activity of the gland will have fallen to about 10 per cent of its original level. As evidence of this inadequacy, immune and autoimmune diseases, such as rheumatism and cancer, appear with increasing frequency.

The regular replacement of thymus hormones can therefore counteract the genesis of diseases of old age and enable the already diseased organism to react in defence. It is also known that zinc deficiency minimises the lymphocyte function in the immune system. Other influences can deplete the immune system and cause a breakdown within the cells. Where there is a lack of the required amino acids, the malignant tissue will further degenerate because of insufficient support resulting from an incomplete protein chain of amino acids.

In our battles to overcome cancer, we hear more and more about possible stimulation of the immune system, which is a powerful and complex defence mechanism for the body to guard itself against foreign matter and invading viruses, bacteria and parasites. If kept in good order, the immune system is equally capable of absorbing and destroying cancer cells. When I have needed to stimulate the complex action of the immune system, I have found *interferon, germanium* and *laetrile* to be invaluable.

Immunity is the degree of resistance that a body can muster to a type of invading microorganism resulting from one or more of these factors: inheritance, an attack of a particular infection, or vaccination or some other artificial means of preventing a disease. Immunity is due to the presence of antibodies. Antibodies are proteins present in the blood and antigens are substances that stimulate the production of antibodies or react with them. Antibodies can originate naturally or spontaneously or be acquired through vaccination etc. Harmful microorganisms, invading the body, act as antigens and stimulate the production of antibodies, which oppose their activities. Antibodies are specific in their reaction, directing it only against a particular kind of microorganism or even a particular strain of it. When an organism invades the body, appropriate antibodies may already exist, and if they are present in adequate amounts, the infected person will not develop the disease.

If a microorganism does invade the body, antibodies to it are produced in about ten days. Once this has taken place, these are likely to remain indefinitely in the blood and may thus prevent a person suffering a second attack of that particular infection. It is therefore unusual for a person to have a second attack of mumps, for example, because there is considerable antibody reaction to this infection; conversely, it is very common for a person to have many attacks of the common cold, to which the antibody reaction is minimal. A child acquires some antibodies from its mother if she has had a particular infection, as these can be transmitted to the child *in utero*. These antibodies can usually prevent a newborn baby from getting that particular infection, but they mostly disappear within a few weeks, leaving the child open to attack.

The weakening of the immune system can be approximately divided into three separate actions or happenings. Initially, there is an enlargement of the adrenal cortex. The hormones produced by this part of the adrenal glands assist the normal body functions in times of stress. In order to produce more hormones to cope with the increased demand, the gland increases in size. If the stress of over-production continues for too long, the gland cannot keep pace and eventually loses its ability to produce enough hormones. Then there is shrinkage in the lymphatic tissue which, as we know, is actively involved with the production of immune cells. A specific type of immune cell may disappear completely from the body as a result. Finally, there may also be ulcerations in the lining of the stomach and the duodenum. These may in themselves be only minor but are, nevertheless, potentially dangerous and even life-threatening.

When foreign matter or antigens manage to invade the body, the immune system responds in a specific way. The humoral response system synthesises and secretes antibodies compatible with the intruding antigen, whilst the cell-mediated immune system responds by making and releasing cells in the particular antigen. The humoral response system acts against bacterial infection and viral re-infections.

The B-lymphocytes play a major role in the immune system and it was not long ago that scientists first managed to separately identify two kinds of lymphocytes, T-cells and B-cells. Each acts separately. It is known that T-cells and B-cells both originate in the bone marrow and nowadays it is also known that the lymphocytes migrate to reach that mature stage.

The macrophages (or scavenger cells) attach themselves to tissue and are transported by the blood. They are on their guard for harmful substances. It is well known that cancer cells will suppress a normal immune system. Tumours often grow in the presence of a defective immune system. Although this growth is a complex process, it is also true that interactions of direct cell contact with oxygen, nutrients, ions and other agents can influence this process. It is, however, equally possible for cancer cells to escape the immune system and establish themselves elsewhere. This means that cancer cells which have escaped destruction have escaped detection by the immune system.

It is important for the immune system that regular detoxification takes place and therefore regular bowel movement is essential. It is sometimes claimed that many cancers originate from the bowels and I always inform relevant patients accordingly. My great-grandmother's advice was that, if necessary, one should use castor oil to avoid any danger of constipation. Fortunately, more palatable means to this end are nowadays available to us.

Often the question arises of how immune damage occurs and here several factors could be relevant. More important to the practitioner, however, is that immune complexes of the appropriate type must be indicated in the tissue or the organ. An accurate assessment of the damage due to immune complex disease is important in order to decide which disease has attacked the immune system. A disease could well result from a minor infection, inhalation of antigenic dust, or ingestion of any unsuitable food or drink. Monitoring the immune system is of great importance and fortunately today we have various types of apparatus and devices which prove helpful in this. The possibility of identifying the cause of any attack on the immune system offers great scope for further research. Since 1950, trials have been continually undertaken to assess how vaccination and immunisation can influence the immune system.

Among its many functions, the thymus gland also forms the hormone peptide. Throughout life, T-lymphocytes are engaged in permanent defensive action, constantly influenced by health and illness. The thymus gland is located under the breastbone, and from there it directs the lymphocytes to where they are needed and deploys them as key operatives in the immune system. Production of lymphocyte cells occurs in the bone marrow, thymus, spleen, tonsils, adenoids and in the lymphoid tissue found in the small intestine.

The soft tissue in the hollows of the long bones of the arms and legs, known as the bone marrow, produces cells which are destined to migrate as they continue to multiply. They progress to become the immuno-commutant, or to produce immunity. Through this intricate 'computerised' mechanism, the lymph nodes also bring together the specialised cooperating functions needed to produce immunity.

Lymph nodes are small, compact structures lying in groups along the course of the lymphatic vessels and this network is comparable to the system of blood vessels. It should therefore be understood that the lymphatic system plays an important preventative and defensive role.

I have already remarked on the fact that the thymus gland slowly shrinks into disappearance as we get older. You may be interested to see the appropriate figures that back up this process: a newborn baby has about 1–1.5 million cells in the thymus; at the age of 20, this will be reduced to 700,000 cells; this figure will have decreased to about 250,000 in a 40-year-old.

Considering the importance of these cells to our immune system, one must agree that any stimulation of these cells is fully justified. Nothing can be done to reverse the shrinking process of the thymus gland, but extra care of all the endocrine glands, specifically the thyroid gland, will not go amiss.

It is no exaggeration to refer to the thymus gland as the 'brain centre' for the whole of the immune system. If this is weak, the body will easily fall prey to viruses and allergies. It has also become generally accepted that if there is a weakening of hormonal reactions, the immune system also suffers. This more or less translates into the requirement that all endocrine glands be in harmony with each other. It has been shown in recent research that not only the thyroid but also the pituitary gland is related closely to the activation of immunoglobulin.

One of my favourite sayings is 'Illness is disharmony'. Anything in the human system that goes out of harmony will cause problems. Could it be a coincidence that the solar spectrum consists of seven basic colours and that there are seven endocrine glands? Never mind how small and insignificant these glands may seem, minor changes can cause either positive or negative deviations.

It has already been mentioned that cancer need not necessarily be caused by physical reasons, but can also be induced by a negative mental attitude. Emotions, stress and trauma greatly influence the endocrine glands. This explains the increasing popularity of holistic medicine. Unfortunately, this approach is still regarded as unorthodox, yet here the patient is treated as a whole and complete being and every aspect of life is studied to obtain a complete picture of him or her. Certain forms of meditation (such as prayer and visualisation techniques) are practised with a view to balancing the endocrine system, which then creates a hormonal balance. Science still has only a limited understanding of the hormonal workings of the endocrine system. It is time that more research was done in that area.

Let us have a look at the pineal gland. There is little doubt that this gland – or the 'third eye' as it is sometimes called – is influenced negatively by stress and positively by prayer and meditation. However, we don't yet know enough about the physical aspect of the pineal gland. This gland, by means of acupuncture, can be balanced. If a patient is under a great deal of stress, working on this particular gland can have very good results.

The pituitary gland is said to be the key to the chemistry of the whole of the body. The pituitary hormones chemically affect the cell membranes. Therefore, the chemical reactions in the body do not work properly when the pituitary gland is in any way impaired or prevented from doing its correct job. A good intake of protein from vegetable rather than animal sources is most important for the production of hormones, and also the different enzymes in the body. If the enzyme production is insufficient, the hormone balance will fail the immune system.

The pituitary gland is often also referred to as the master gland or conductor of the endocrine orchestra, and it releases hormones to either promote or inhibit the release of other endocrine hormones. Indirectly, it controls such basic processes as rate of growth, metabolic rate, water and electrolyte balance, kidney filtration, ovulation and lactation. It responds to hormones released by the region of the brain known as the hypothalamus and is a physical link between the nervous and the endocrine systems.

The thyroid is a glandular link between the brain and the reproductive organs and it is certain that the thyroid can be triggered or inhibited by emotional disturbances, directly influencing circulation, respiration, tissue growth and repair. Overproduction of thyroxine from the thyroid gland will lead to problems and, equally, so will underproduction. We often see how individuals are emotionally affected when a defect appears.

The pancreas secretes digestive enzymes into the small intestine, which produces hormones for release into the blood. The digestive enzymes are crucial because the incorrect breakdown of ingested fats, proteins and sugars can lead to digestive complaints, e.g. diabetes or hypoglycaemia. The islets of Langerhans – a group of cells within the pancreas – secrete insulin into the blood and so influence the level of glucose in the body. The pancreas also plays an important role in regulating the hormonal balance.

When we realise that the adrenals produce 50 different natural steroid hormones, we recognise the importance of these glands. Some of these hormones are involved in the conversion of dietary protein and fat into glucose, while others suppress inflammation and promote healing. Yet another group regulates the blood/iron balance in the kidneys and still others affect the sex functions. The principal hormone produced, called adrenaline, is ready to respond to any emergencies –

The gonads – the male and female sexual endocrine glands – are for the reproduction of the species. At puberty, the hormones aid development of the secondary sexual characteristics of the male and female bodies and activate their reproductive systems. One of the roles of the gonads is harmonising all the endocrine glands. We see too often in cases of stress or menopausal problems that these glands play an enormous role, physically as well as mentally. It is well known that poor nutrition affects the sexual glands and that the functions of the vital organs will be impaired if the diet is lacking proper nutrition. All in all, it is clear that these apparently insignificant and small glands have an enormous effect on the well-being of the immune system. Overall healthcare is therefore extremely important.

I have already touched upon whether it could be a coincidence that there are seven endocrine glands and seven basic colours in the solar spectrum. It is, however, a fact that the eye possesses seven layers of light receptors. Through these, the cosmic force of the seven basic colours influences the endocrine glands. Because of the depressive aspect of the illness, a cancer patient can therefore turn this cosmic force to their advantage, focusing on getting better. The seven layers of light receptors in the retina of the eye allow practitioners of iridology to quickly detect disturbances. How sensitive these receptors are is clearly noticeable from observing cancer patients who overindulge in watching television, as this can cause disharmony.

Generally, awareness is growing of the adverse effects of computer screens, word processors, television screens, etc. Often coordination problems result from overexposure to these and further study on this aspect would be beneficial. By no means am I implying that these screens are the cause of cancer; what I am saying is that one should remain cautious, as they can cause some disharmony in the body.

Each case of immune deficiency should be judged individually, as the immune system can be influenced in so many ways. When I saw the lady I mentioned at the beginning of this chapter I was intrigued to know how she was still alive 38 years on, as she had been extremely ill. At that time, I had advised her about certain remedies, possible lifestyle changes and dietary management. I could see that she had a terrific will to live. She wanted to be with her husband and take care of her children, and she told me that every day she visualised that she would get better. I taught her some helpful exercises and prescribed several vitamins, minerals and trace elements. In particular, I gave her *Petasan*, *Petasites* capsules and beta carotene, and she kept going. I saw her for over a year, during which time she improved and the hospital even told her that she was doing very well. It is a real joy to see how well she is today. She is living proof that cancer can be beaten and that real benefits can be achieved from having a positive attitude. Success stories such as this give me such pleasure. Often the secret with illness and disease is to be able to rebuild the immune system. This lady's immune system had been almost non-existent, but she said jubilantly that she was so grateful she had come to me, as I had helped her beat cancer through complementary methods, in conjunction with her orthodox treatment.

Today, I again pondered on immunity and how it really works. My great Dutch friend, Marie-Louise Schicht, whom I have known for many years, said a few wise things about the immune system. She said that the immune system is really the defence system of our body. Part of this is the lymphatic system, which is a net of lymphatic vessels similar to the layout of the blood vessels in our organism. From every part of our body, toxic substances are transported via these lymphatic vessels to the smaller and larger lymph nodes, which are the 'sewage plants' of the organism. Bacteria, toxins, alien substances and waste products from the body itself, like dead cells and bacteria, are transported to these detoxification centres.

Some substances, e.g. those from cow's milk and certain fats, are sent directly from the intestines via the small lymphatic vessels situated in the intestinal wall, to the main centre of the lymphatic defence system situated in the abdomen. There, and in the other lymph nodes, such as the tonsils and the appendix, the substances mentioned above are cleaned and detoxified. After this, all waste materials which cannot be used are taken up by the venous blood and eliminated. The most important organs through which this elimination of toxins takes place are the skin, the kidneys, the lungs and the intestines. As the greatest dangers that threaten our health develop in the abdomen, most lymphatic vessels and lymph nodes are found there. Here also a very important substance for our defence, immunoglobulin, is produced. Every second, no matter how slight the danger, millions of defensive cells are used and have to be replaced over and over again. The spleen and the thyroid gland are also an important part of this defence system.

Hundreds of years ago, physicians already knew that there were many interactions between the outer skin and the inner mucous membrane which could be made use of therapeutically. There are people who have a so-called 'lymphatic constitution'. These people very often become ill when their lymphatic defences have been weakened. They then suffer from health problems such as the common cold or a sore throat, which are nothing but a simple defence reaction of the body. Such natural reactions always have a purpose and serve to eliminate toxins.

When the health of the organism is at risk, the immune system will automatically react. One can understand this best by observing the simple defensive reactions that happen every day: if dust gets into the nose, we sneeze in order to get rid of it and protect our respiratory tract. Coughing, clearing the throat and sneezing sometimes have a double purpose – they help not only to dispose of dust particles but also to eliminate the accumulated mucous. If something gets into the eyes, tears will clean them. If we have eaten some food that does not agree with us, we get diarrhoea or we have to vomit. The main purpose of this is always the cleansing of the organism. Simple health problems will be cured by simple measures. The organism will fight greater health problems by using a variety of stronger defensive measures.

A lymphatic constitution is sometimes hereditary, but it is also possible to acquire such a constitution during the course of life. This can start when one is still young, for example when small children eat too many sweets or drink cow's milk. In this case, the tonsils or the lymph nodes in the neck start to swell as the organism tries to neutralise the toxins. If it is not possible to neutralise all the toxins, the child may get tonsillitis (inflammation of the tonsils). It will depend upon the physician and the parents if this inflammation is treated in the correct way, by natural means, or if the child will suffer all its life from lymphatic diseases. An operation to remove the tonsils or treatment with antibiotics may have serious consequences, as the tonsils can no longer act as a defensive organism. After some time, other parts of the lymphatic system, such as the bronchial tubes or the mucous membranes of the sinuses, will take over those defensive functions which formerly were the task of the tonsils. If this happens and the person in question still eats an unhealthy diet, these secondary defensive systems will also become overstrained. Then chronic diseases of the bronchial system and the sinuses, as well as serious diseases of the abdomen, may develop.

Our immune system nowadays has to work non-stop at full power and is constantly overstressed. Its cells die by the million and cannot be replaced quickly enough. Innumerable alien substances, which have no place in the human body, prevent normal body functions. Any substance entering our digestive tract that cannot be used in some way means needless work for the immune system and a waste of energy.

We live in a world full of harmful substances, toxins, microbes and other tiny creatures, and each day many of these penetrate our body. Most of the time, such alien elements are rendered harmless by our defensive mechanism and are eliminated as soon as possible. But as long as all symptoms are suppressed through drugs regardless of the number of casualties, there will be more and more chronic illness in the world.

Your immune system is your private army for battling disease and generally defending your body against countless intruders. This army is made up of battalions of cells with varying skills and numerous 'bases' and 'factories' for the supply of ammunition. If the 'soldiers', the cells, are weak and unhealthy, or if the factories are short of raw materials, then the army is likely to lose the battle. If the army is in good condition and well equipped, then it will usually be able to fight off anything from the common cold to cholera or cancer. The basic cause of many illnesses is the poor condition of the sick person's 'army' – this is called a depressed immune system. Getting the immune system into good order will often overcome the illness. If a nation loses a war with another nation, it is not simply because it was attacked; it loses because its own army is not strong enough to defeat the invaders.

A depressed immune system is recognised as the direct cause of allergic conditions such as asthma and eczema. The condition of the immune system will, however, also affect all other illnesses, from how quickly a burn or fracture heals, to how effectively a virus such as cholera is beaten off. An experiment with very healthy volunteers on highly nutritious diets found that all of them, when put in contact with the cholera virus, were able to fight it off quickly and easily. They did not actually contract full-blown cholera because their immune systems were in excellent working order. It can be seen, therefore, that the cause of an illness is not just the existence of a condition such as a nasty bug, but is more often an immune system that is not up to the job of fighting it off.

There are two quite different ways of dealing with an illness: the symptom treatment approach and the cause treatment approach. Unfortunately, symptom treatment is the most common approach today because most medical research is funded by pharmaceutical companies that can make fortunes by treating symptoms, but nothing very much by getting to the cause! You will soon see why.

Taking the example of cancer, symptom treatment would involve attacking the cancer cells directly in order to get rid of them. This involves such methods as surgery, chemotherapy and irradiation. Cancers, however, are developing in our bodies most of the time – a healthy immune system will quite easily keep the cancer cells in check and destroy them. Cancer is a condition that only gets out of hand when the immune system is in poor working order. You can see now that it is actually the depressed immune system that is causing the illness. Cause treatment, on the other hand, would try to build up the immune system so that it could resume its work of battling with the invaders.

Of course, symptom treatment does have a place in good medical practice, but usually as an emergency treatment while the cause is being dealt with. Getting at the cause and cleaning up the root problems tends to take longer, but cause treatment must be implemented if the person is to become really well. For example, a cancer tumour may need to be surgically removed, but if the patient's immune system is not rebuilt to a healthy state, the body is likely to succumb to other cancers.

Symptom treatment often appears to give instant results – a painkiller, for example, will cut off the pain message to the brain, so that it will seem as though the problem has gone away. Of course, it hasn't. The body is still undergoing the shock and trauma of whatever is actually happening to cause the pain, even though the brain is not processing the information. Believing otherwise would be like being a commanding officer who, while the battle is going against him, shoots his own messengers and then celebrates a victory on the basis that no one has told him that he has lost. The cause of the pain is not being dealt with by the painkiller. Another example is the drugs used to stop the spasms of an asthmatic lung – these can be a valuable emergency measure, but do nothing to rid the body of the asthma, so that further attacks can always be expected. Yet, asthma can be cured.

Clearly there is a place for symptom treatment, but it must not be in any way confused with cause treatment or be thought of as getting at the cause. The effects of cause treatment can be positive and permanent. It usually has the benefit of no side effects, making you feel better and better with time, whereas 'symptom' treatment usually exacerbates the problem and makes you feel worse and worse with time. Cause treatment also has the benefit of being cheaper in the long run and of giving you the ability to take control of the problem yourself. It is sometimes fear of taking control oneself that worries people with little self-confidence and makes them want to leave it all to someone else. Don't be afraid! You can enjoy the challenge and you will find that you are not alone in the fight.

Let us return to the function of the immune system. When it is being attacked, the body releases a very powerful and toxic substance called histamine, which is probably the most deadly of its weapons. An antidote to this histamine, called antihistamine, is produced by the liver to protect our cells from being damaged by this substance. Not having the antihistamine would be a bit like conducting chemical warfare without wearing protective clothing yourself! If there isn't enough antihistamine to counteract all the histamine (perhaps the liver is under par, or the siege is just too great), the body does all it can to clear the toxins from itself in other ways. Some bodies try to get rid of it by passing it back out through the nearest mucous membrane, which becomes inflamed, as with the lungs in asthmatics or the sinuses with sufferers of hay fever. Most people's bodies try to deal with the problem in less obvious ways which can have long-term and very nasty effects.

An important aspect of the warfare is, therefore, the rubbish it produces. The ability of your body to clean up the mess will have a great effect on how well you conduct the next battle. A cluttered and putrefying battlefield would not be very effective! Another source of 'rubbish' is the by-products of our bodies burning food as fuel. Our bodies need vast amounts of energy to carry out all the chemical and physical work necessary to keep us alive. The release of energy by oxidation means that the electrons, which are tiny parts orbiting in each atom, leave the atom in singles and in pairs. It is like a fire with sparks flying off. The atoms which fly off with one atom 'hole' are called free radicals. A stable atom has its electrons all paired off – the negative-charged ones with the positive-charged ones. However, a free radical has one spare electron which gives the atom an electrical charge, so it goes off looking for something to attach to. There are those that fly off to do special jobs, mostly to do with the respiratory system and enzyme activity.

If the fuel is poor quality or contaminated, however, various species of dangerous free radicals are produced. These can wreak havoc by attaching to stable molecules and turning them into erratic free radicals as well. A healthy body will be able to screen these free radicals and keep them under control. Most often, however, the body taking in poor fuel is also likely to have poor health, including a poor screening process. It is rather like having a screen in front of a fire to hold the sparks in check. If there are holes in the screen, or there are so many sparks that the screen is knocked over, the protection will be lost.

Free radicals going haywire cause havoc which is called 'oxy-stress'. This stress mostly influences the state of the immune system and is a major factor in the ageing process. The most common form of free radical harm is from poor quality (that is, refined and processed) or rancid oils and fats. This is called lipid peroxidation and is thought to be a major factor in most age-related diseases such as arthritis, dementia and many cancers.

Your body has two lines of defence to protect itself from free radicals and oxy-stress. The first is 'free radical scavengers', special enzymes whose job it is to protect other molecules from free radicals. These include superoxide dismutase (SOD), glutathione and catalase. The second line of defence is antioxidant nutrients – we get these through food. They act like mops to soak up the free radicals and take them out of the body. These include vitamins C, A and E, selenium and amino acids such as methione, taurine, cysteine and L-glutamine.

The free radicals present in our body should be the productive ones that result from burning quality food in a well-controlled way. These days, however, there are many other sources of free radicals, such as radiations of many kinds (e.g. electromagnetic fields from overhead power lines), pollutants such as ozone, nitrogen dioxide, sulphur dioxide, cigarette smoke, solvents, pesticides, drugs, and heavy metal poisoning by lead, cadmium and aluminium. This heavy bombardment of volatile free radicals makes it all the more important that the diet is wholesome, in order to provide lines of defence and protection. Because the level of bombardment is so unnaturally high, it is often necessary to supplement the diet with antioxidant nutrients to combat the free radicals. Antioxidant nutrients are major weapons in any immune system-related illness.

With such an amazingly complex immune system, with all its inbuilt safeguards, what could possibly go wrong? Two of the things that affect your army are the strength and effectiveness of the fortress walls and the size and strength of the foe.

Let us examine each of these in turn. Looking at the strength and effectiveness of the fortress walls – the fortress walls are the first line of defence you have against intruders trying to get into your body. These include the skin and the mucous linings of the digestive tract, genitals, lungs, nasal passages, etc. These surface areas not only have their own battalions of specialist soldiers and defence systems, but also usually use parasitic but 'friendly' bacteria to help in the defence. Bacteria that are not friendly allies are always also resident in these areas, but are kept in check by the friendly bacteria. There are therefore two aspects to keeping the fortress walls effective: the cells making up the different components of the walls themselves and their specialist armies must be kept in good condition; and the friendly bacteria must also be kept in good condition. Hay fever is a good example of what can happen when the fortress walls are not in good condition. It is thought that when the mucous lining of the nasal passages is in poor condition, the cells are not as tightly knit together as they should be.

Looking at the size and strength of the foe – the idea of cutting down on the numbers of intruders to the body is not new. Everyday hygiene aims to do this. Our problem is more often that we don't recognise the enemy. It's very difficult to catch anything from your cat or dog, yet you are more likely to be concerned about washing your hands after patting them than you would be about intruders from your favourite soap or chemical deodorant. These latter items, however, are likely to provide you with both numerous bacteria (which the healthy body should deal with fairly easily) and chemical toxins (which your body will find much more difficult to handle). It is estimated that, on average, each person in Britain consumes about 2 kg of chemical pollutants each year. Considering that even a trace of most chemicals can have profound effects, especially on the immune system, this adds up to a major attack. A body in optimum health with a good supply of a wide range of nutrients should be able to detoxify a fair proportion of this, so if you have to live in a city and be subject to petrol pollution, for example, you can minimise the damage.

I would recommend that everyone – but especially those people with evidence of already depressed immune systems – reduce the scale of the attack by measures such as the following:

> ● Use only the simplest cleaning agents around the house and always environmentally friendly ones, because these will be friendlier to your body too. Never use disinfectants (especially around children) and never use sprays of any sort, whether polish or perfume, etc.
> ● Cut down on the amount of plastic in the environment as much as possible because plastics constantly give off a faint gas. This includes children's toys, lunch boxes, plastic food containers and plastic food wraps, plastic work surfaces, synthetic carpets, foam pillows, etc.

● Be aware of and minimise your contact with items that are clearly based on chemicals that permeate your environment easily. Examples in this category would be many marker pens, glues and solvents.

● Keep the home and work environment well ventilated.

● Use only the simplest natural body-care products, in moderation. Definitely no antiperspirants, medicated products or sterilising agents, as these are very damaging. Let your skin breathe properly. Do not wash so often that your skin is oil-free and unable to manufacture vitamin D from sunlight. The way you smell will have more to do with your state of health, stress levels, skin activity and what is going on inside you than with the amount of washing that you do. Genital and excretory areas should be cleansed with nothing more than clear warm water, unless there is any indication of irritation, in which case live yoghurt could be effective. The use of tampons and vaginal cleansers or deodorants of any kind is extremely unwise. Toxic shock syndrome is only one of the possible effects of using them.

● Clothing that is next to the skin, in particular, must allow your skin to breathe, and should therefore be made of natural fibres. Ideally, these would not contain dyes such as the bright white dioxin, but this is a lot to hope for at the moment! Children's clothing really should be all natural. Clothing should be washed with the simplest fragrance-free ecological cleaning agents and be thoroughly rinsed. So many people have obvious allergies to what is in or on the clothes they wear that it is clear most of us must be affected in some lesser way. Chemicals from synthetic fibres, from dyes and from cleaning agents will most likely (though perhaps not obviously) cause constant battles at a first line of defence – the skin. This unnecessarily depletes valuable resources from the whole army's reserves, while not doing much for the beauty of the skin itself.

● Most importantly, cut out pollutants taken internally,

in both food and as much as possible in medications. 'Fast' sugars and caffeine, like most drugs, are very debilitating polluters. The fungicides, hormones, artificial fertilisers and other chemical pollutants in non-organically farmed fruit and vegetables make up a very nasty enemy. This chemically farmed produce also tends to supply very little in the way of nutrients which would help to combat the ill effects of the pollutants. Certainly, vitamin C is rare! Meeting this goal would be the most effective measure for working towards optimum good health. Among other things, most meat and processed foods are major sources of internal pollution. It should also be remembered that pollutants from within factories, especially from cleaning agents, are likely to be present in processed foods. A friend of mine worked in a famous brewery, where he nightly donned something resembling a spacesuit and entered enormous metal vats where he sprayed a highly toxic cleaning agent. The vats were used to make beer the next day without any attempt to even rinse them out.

● Most drugs and medications are very taxing on the immune system – and most other body systems. Avoid unnatural painkillers, such as aspirin and paracetamol, tranquillisers, barbiturates, etc. Find truly helpful ways to meet your needs. Question any medication your doctor suggests – you have a right to do this – and aim for an understanding of exactly what is going on, so that you can work towards cause rather than symptom treatment.

HOW THE IMMUNE SYSTEM IS AFFECTED BY STRESS

When your body has demands placed upon it which exceed your resources to adjust to the demands, the nervous system answers with stress responses. The chemical pathways of these stress responses tend to use many parts of the body which are also crucial to the immune system, so it is not surprising that conditions of one system will affect the other.

CANCER AND THE IMMUNE SYSTEM

The adrenalin you tend to feel as a 'rush' or a 'high' is an attempt to get you ready for a 'fight or flight' situation. This hypes you up with a faster pulse, faster breathing and other effects you can't see or feel. You can't feel any of the effects of the corticosteroids, but they have a tremendous impact on the immune system. One corticosteroid called cortisol (also called hydrocortisone) will degrade the tissues of the thymus gland and lymph nodes, and increase T-suppressor cells, while decreasing T-helper cells and interfere with the production of the natural killer cells and interferon. The realisation that high cortisol levels exacerbate immune system-related diseases has made cortisol-lowering drugs a new field of major research. A number of drugs have been found effective in chronic diseases because they lowered the cortisol in the blood. The problem with these drugs is, of course, their other side effects. But there is a powerful *natural* cortisol-lowering drug without side effects, which the body loves to draw on if it can get enough in a sound diet. This is vitamin C!

Physical stresses, such as lack of sleep, usually lead to emotional stresses such as irritability. You can see now why emotional stresses – which range from constant negative or worrying thoughts, through to depression and anger, to major bereavement (such as the loss of a spouse or child) – will also affect the immune system and increase the chance of disease. This is why love and support for someone during an illness makes an enormous difference to how that person pulls through the illness. It is why sensible stress management in the workplace leads to less illness and greater opportunity to achieve. It is also why hurts, such as bereavement, need to be brought into the open and dealt with lovingly. It is not uncommon for one spouse to die of general poor health soon after the death of the other.

Like all the other systems in your body, the nervous system needs building blocks to produce, repair and generally run smoothly. It wants to be able to adjust well to different situations and crises. So, a healthy person with a sound system based on good building blocks will deal, for example, with a major bereavement much more effectively than if they were in poorer health. The shock of being in an accident will bring on cancer where the seatbelt struck the breast only if the person's general health and therefore nervous and immune systems are under par. Someone I knew died under such circumstances three months after an accident. She was 30 years old. She ate a typical 'egg and chips' diet with few nutrients and plenty of pollutants. Her immune system was not equipped to cope with the shock of the accident.

It is encouraging to know that your health – and the health of those you love – is not a matter entirely out of your hands. You can do an enormous amount to influence susceptibility to disease and the ability to cope with stress.

There are five aspects to building up the immune system:

- You need to change to a wholesome diet.
- You need to exercise regularly, preferably including at least 20 minutes of aerobic exercise, and get at least half an hour of sunshine daily (not necessarily direct sunshine).
- You need to carry out detoxification, as detailed earlier in the book.
- You need to deal with the stresses in your life.
- You need to supplement your diet with a suitable range of nutrients. Each person's needs are individual and would be best catered for by consulting a naturopath or dietary consultant to devise a programme specifically for you. Before doing so, you should consult your GP if you are on any medication or if you have any specific disease or illness.

The following is a simple, straightforward, safe, nutritional programme that provides high levels of a correct spectrum of nutrients for boosting the immune system. You should take them all:

- Antioxidant nutrients in a tablet form, containing minerals, amino acids and vitamins which are all noted for free radical scavenging and stimulating the immune system. Follow the dosage instructions on the container.

● Multivitamins and minerals in a tablet form, containing an extensive range of nutrients and a well-balanced range of B vitamins. Try and look for tablets without the addition of iron if you are already ill. Again, follow the dosage instructions on the container.

● GLA – these capsules provide omega-6 polyunsaturated gamma linoleic acid. Especially necessary when quality oils and fats are not a part of the diet. Follow the dosage instructions on the container.

This is just a basic, though well-rounded guide. You must, however, allow three months for beneficial results. When you begin this programme, there may be signs of withdrawal (such as headaches) and cleansing (such as skin eruptions, body odour and different types of stools). However, once you have taken the time to understand and practise the principles, you will adapt quite easily.

A number of nature's products have been found to help stimulate the immune system in a positive way. The substance generally recognised as the most powerful immune stimulant and restorative is called *Lentinan*. It, and similar glucose substances, is found in the medical grade of the Japanese shitake and reishi mushrooms respectively. These can be bought as a powder to be taken as one teaspoonful daily, or two teaspoonfuls in the case of AIDS or cancer. These mushrooms, which have been used both as food and medicinally for a very long time in the Orient, have active principles which have been shown experimentally to be anticancer, antiviral and cholesterol-lowering. The reishi has been used very effectively against chronic asthmatic bronchitis.

Echinacea is a herb which Western and American Indian herbalists have used for a very long time for disorders relating to the immune system. Laboratory studies have confirmed that *echinacea* raises the white blood cell count and induces photocytosis, which means the white cells increase their activities in gobbling and digesting unfriendly aliens. Many experiments and efforts have been made to isolate the factors within *echinacea* which have immune-stimulating properties. Its effectiveness, however, turns back on itself as doses get higher, after somewhere between one and three grams are taken, so it is best to stay under one gram. The herbal tablet *Immuno* contains nine grams in each tablet, so I recommend that only one be taken daily unless you are already very ill. Do not double up on *echinacea* if you are taking herbs for different reasons, such as for immune-building and for a skin disorder. *Echinaforce* from Bioforce has been shown to be one of the best in the world!

Perhaps the most accessible and certainly an extremely powerful immune stimulant and natural bactericide is the humble garlic. Its properties are so many that research papers about garlic are coming out about every 20 days. Studies have shown that it has powerful properties for directly destroying bacteria and fungi, and inhibits viral multiplication. Even the HIV virus, the precursor of AIDS, finds it difficult to grow in a garlic medium in tissue culture in the laboratory. It has been effectively used in the prevention of intestinal parasites, cancer of the digestive organs and meningitis. It has now been shown, however, that garlic is able to do more than just kill microorganisms like a safer version of an antibiotic. It also actively stimulates the immune system, especially macrophage and B-lymphocyte activity. Laboratory-isolated killer cells from garlic-eating people have been found to be much more capable of destroying tumours than the same type of cell from non-garlic consumers. Garlic is powerful and, as a supplement, should be consumed carefully, preferably with food and at intervals. There are a number of garlic supplements for those who do not eat much in their food, including the 'odourless' version.

In order to boost the immune system further, there are some very worthwhile steps that can be taken which have the added benefit of aiding relaxation. There are various training courses, self-help groups, psychological approaches, supportive nursing care and counselling available. We must not forget about healing of the mind, which is so important, as we all know that the mind is the strongest part of the body. In the next chapter, I shall speak about a method of self-healing which, through meditation and visualisation, with the addition of a positive attitude, can prove that the mind is stronger than the body and that the spirit or the soul might well be the key to improving our health.

Chapter Eight

Cancer and the Mind

I have often said in lectures and during consultations with patients that a cancer cell is like a brain cell. It is quite interesting to see the extent to which cancer is influenced by the mind, both positively and negatively. Through visualisation techniques, meditation and positive thinking, a cancer patient can survive longer or, even more amazingly, beat cancer entirely.

All cancers are related to the liver. Even if cancer develops in another part of the body – such as the breast, lung, stomach, etc. – the liver is always involved. Therefore, while it is important that we see cancer as a metabolic problem, it is also important to know that the liver is often responsible when a cancer patient becomes depressed and, again, dietary management plays an enormous role here.

I was greatly encouraged when I read Professor Michael Gearin-Tosh's book *The Living Proof*, in which he emphasises the terrific benefits he obtained from the breathing exercises I recommended to him. Those exercises (which I shall go into further in the last part of this chapter) are of ultimate importance in creating a positive mind, positive action and positive influence on cancer cells. One must not forget that, in a nutshell, cancer is cells that are out of control and the more holistically we see a patient, the more overall benefits he or she will obtain.

We have not one but three bodies – physical, mental and

emotional. Healing of the mind plays an enormous role in our overall health and it is therefore necessary to seriously examine this subject in order to understand that a good mental attitude is very important. Genuine healing by the power of the mind rests upon a very solid foundation of principles. The force of nature is much stronger than anybody thinks. It is quite amazing how strong the mind is, something we find when we look at people who have developed a strong positive attitude by finding a true remedy for almost every ill of the body, the mind and environment, and the power to conquer life and its problems.

I once spent a whole day with Uri Geller, when we took part in lectures together. Although I was always very sceptical about his work, while he was demonstrating with the aid of several objects, I could see by the enormous concentration he displayed that there was nothing gimmicky about what he was doing – it was simply that he had discovered the secret of the strong powers that the mind has to overcome terrific problems. Before he performed a certain exercise, he produced a few packets of Brussels sprout seeds that he had bought that day and, as proof, showed me the receipt from the shop where he had made his purchase. He said he wanted to show me something. He took one packet of the seeds, placed it in the palm of his hand and told the seeds to grow. Almost instantly, those seeds began to sprout. Then he asked four children from the audience for their help. He gave the children some seeds from the same packet, asked them to place the seeds in the palms of their hands and to shout at the seeds that they should grow and, again, within seconds, they grew. He repeated the demonstration with the second packet of seeds and it was amazing to see that those seeds also sprouted. In other words, he had used his positive mind to tell them to grow – and it worked. It wasn't a trick; it was a straightforward exercise to show how powerful the mind is.

Each time public interest in the subject of our hidden mental powers is aroused, the popularity of mental methods of healing spreads rapidly. This has nothing to do with *spiritual* healing. It is simply the ability to develop one's own mind so it can become capable of producing a strong positive action. Science has conclusively demonstrated in its analyses that the body wants to be healed. It has a healing power within itself that needs to be exercised, as most of our brain is not used and lies idle. There are several methods that can be employed here but, regardless of what method is used, it is purely a question of developing this positive action by exercising the mind, which will become an active healing force once it has been unlocked. I find this so important with cancer patients and I am therefore totally in favour of helping cancer patients who have lost all hope to employ visualisation, prayer and meditation as a daily exercise.

We often become slaves, dependent on methods or remedies that ignore the mind, and we possibly have greater faith in methods and remedies than in ourselves. We must not forget that the mind is stronger than the body and that in the physical structure of human beings, the mind is the basis of complete harmony between mind, body and soul. It is a fundamental principle that light and gravity exist – and have always existed – like the immense quantities of electricity that have been present in the atmosphere since the beginning of time and which, although invisible, are like the spiritual light that exists and of which we are all part.

The cynic might say, 'I don't believe in Creation, because how could God have created the earth on the first day, when He instructed there should be light and there was light whilst, on the fourth day, He created the moon, the stars and the sun?' To the same cynics, there is one answer – God had a much more important light, that being the spiritual light which he created on the first day. If we discover that light and walk in it, then we have a part in the almighty power that God will give to us to keep in contact with the great powers that He will freely give. While modern science might increasingly demonstrate the present power and possibility of unseen forces, the basic reality lies in the fact that the spiritual light created by God on the first day is the most important factor in healing oneself. We must have a harmonious contact with the giver of all life.

There are a lot of patients who become incurable because they have not discovered the great power of that light. That force will be present forever. If one changed the key and the atoms, the whole thing would fall apart. Scientifically, we can prove a lot, but in a simple way, accepting that great gift of God will help us realise the power of the mind over the physical body. This understanding comes naturally and doesn't need a lot of education. There may be large groups who, in an academic way, try to discover this divine process, but the basic fact is that we must learn to accept it as a child might and must humbly ask the Creator to help us develop this strong power of belief in our own mind and to overcome all the ignorance, fears, doubts, gloom and passions in finding these God-given powers and realising that they exist within us.

It is simply a matter of considering the remarkable results that can be obtained when we find the silent self-acting healing powers within ourselves. After all, our entire structure – physical, mental, spiritual and emotional – is totally dependent on the principle of our reality. Perfect health of mind and body exists only when harmony is found between the three bodies. Health is the primary state of human existence and of natural law.

When we become more conscious of this principle, we enter into a much deeper consciousness which is spiritual yet based on reality, because it is basically the principle of life. It is wonderful when we become a spiritual being in the likeness of the principle of Creation, for the soul is a divine conception of God's own pure idea to create us in his own image and therefore it should be whole, complete and perfect. That higher view of humankind may be difficult to grasp, but it is written in the oldest book, the Bible. It is a wonderful thought that although we are a minute part of Creation, we are still part of it. Similarly, if we take one drop out of the ocean, it is still part of that ocean, and when we put that drop back in the ocean, it is also still part of it. We might just be a drop in the ocean of Creation but we still belong to it, although our bodies might give up. Spiritually, we are part of that great universe that makes us all unique. It is our privilege to discover that spiritual self which is such a help when facing life's battles. The fundamental truth that the spiritual being is always well is of great help in understanding our Creator in His almighty power. We are part of Him and He will always look after us and unite our body, mind and soul if we keep in contact with our spiritual reality.

FEMALE CANCERS

I like the expression 'holistic medicine' because that is really what medicine is all about. Although most doctors are trained only to treat symptoms, it is more beneficial to focus on the cause of the problem. We have not only to treat one body, but three – mental, physical and emotional. Disease and pain often have a mental origin. Thousands of experimental tests have been carried out on this topic and they clearly demonstrate that the human system in its entirety is the instrument of the mind. As I often say, 'The mind directs the body; the body does not direct the mind.' This is demonstrated in the story of Queen Marie Antoinette, whose hair turned white overnight during the bloodbath of the French Revolution. We often find that with people who experience anger, grief, jealousy, work resentment, greed and fear, all these particularly negative influences can poison the mind to such an extent that the body is out of harmony.

If there is a state of mental confusion and the whole body is out of harmony, it can certainly influence the development of cancer cells. Sickness, although often traceable to an abnormal mental state, is due more often to a *subconscious* mental cause than to the state of the conscious mind. Although the mind is one unit, it is dual in its action. It benefits from objective thinking – ideas and pictures in our mind of a false concept will cause a confused mental state and, although nature will attempt to correct this, it will affect the entire human system. When the conscious mind interferes with nature's normal processes through negative or confused thoughts, the subconscious mind will be influenced, so the more positive we are the better. To positively influence the conscious mind will, in turn, influence the subconscious mind and lead to a deeper harmony that will be of benefit to whatever treatment is undertaken.

I often see this with cancer patients who are positive – even with some I thought would not survive. They take positive action, say to themselves that they want to live, to be with their families, their husbands and their children, to enjoy life and get the best out of it. They are often great survivors. Then there are others who I would probably give a greater chance of survival, but if their minds are filled with negative thoughts, it is difficult to plant the seed in their minds that they will get better. Others who totally accept the situation and say they are going to die anyway usually die more quickly. Fighting a disease is a question of having a positive mind and trying to overcome the problem as much as possible. We see this in Professor Michael Gearin-Tosh's book, *The Living Proof*, when he talks of the years he survived by refusing to accept the situation. He fought his own illness and, today, he remains victorious.

There is an interesting quote in the *British Medical Journal* (January 1896): 'Disease of the body is so much influenced by the mind that in each case we have to understand the patient quite as much as the malady.' This is often the case, for we must influence the mind and body positively. The slightest mental activity creates a definite anatomical change. It is said that the imagination is one of the most effective agents which can modify the conditions of health and disease. To actively think that not only are we physical, but spiritual and divinely created in the image and likeness of God, will be of great help in developing a positive mindset that refuses to accept illness or disease. A long time ago, I attended a lecture given by a professor who spoke on cancer. She said that when she woke up in the morning, the first thing she used to do was to greet her husband by saying, 'Good morning, John.' Now she says, 'Good morning, cells, you have kept me alive.' It is much better to be positive, as our thoughts have an impact at a cellular level. We are affected by thought all the time and if a positive thought is strongly cemented in the brain, it will produce positive action. Flowers, animals, trees, mountains and stars are all part of the universal mind. It is wonderful that through the power of our mind, we can govern the strife in our body.

The quality of our thinking is completely dependent on the level of our understanding. Right thoughts are mental pictures that we form of the realities of life – the good, the true and the beautiful. Wrong thoughts are those mental images we form from the evils, wrongs and perversions of life. We will gain a true understanding of life if we learn to differentiate between the true and the false. I learned a lot when I carried out my prison work throughout Britain – for instance, how easily a person can become a criminal when a negative thought becomes cemented in the mind, so that even when that individual is doing wrong, he thinks he is doing right. It is sad to think that negative thoughts can lead to such negative actions. It does not take a lot of effort to educate ourselves to do what is right; we simply need to be able to differentiate between good and evil. We need to have a vision of what is right, for as the Old Book says, 'When there is no vision, the people must perish.' Working on ourselves and trying to do what is right can only benefit our body.

I saw this once with a famous singer who was facing death from a very aggressive cancer. He took a careful look at his life and rid himself of all the excess baggage: everything that he thought was wrong, he replaced with positive actions. Yes, this man was blessed – and his body benefited remarkably from his positive actions. He often said to me that he was so happy he had followed my advice.

The body wants to be healthy. It is a normal state established by nature and the mind has the power to generate this in abundance. In fact, it is almost impossible for a disease to develop when the law of right thinking is fully employed in life. Unfortunately, we often see that when we get depressed and give up the battle, our health deteriorates. Sadly, we cannot always manage to overcome the aggressive nature of some cancers, which can be such that they take over.

Visualising getting better is often of great help. In true healing – which means making whole, strong and perfect – we exercise the higher power that rules mind and spirit. Mathematics is an exercise of numbers and the application must firstly be considered before the correct answer is found. The same goes for health and healing. It is essential to firstly express the will to gain control over the mind. In so doing, control over the body will be achieved.

From a mental image of health, we can see ourselves in our mind's eye as striving for perfection. It is often a good idea to sit down in a peaceful place and say to yourself, 'I will get better, I want to be well, I want to be part of that great ocean of love and although I might be just a little drop in it, I still belong to it.' This can be achieved with quiet meditation and prayer.

When we form a new energy, harmony and wholeness, the gates

will open to enable us to find our inner selves and to realise how unique everyone is. Life and health are important. We have to learn that truly potent healing is the result of the great, infinite love that we can all experience. Potentially, we are capable of more than we realise. In our mind's eye, we have to focus on the development of the soul. The application of the law of healing is right there in our consciousness and when the mind is centred and in harmony, we can achieve more than we thought possible.

Thinking of what is real and perfect will bring about the most wholesome mental changes. By following that direction, we will find that we can overcome disease and ill health to a great extent. The mind is much stronger than we think. I often see this when I manage to get patients to stop thinking about their illness all the time and try to divert their mind in another direction. Then the simple act of thinking becomes so different. Sometimes I say to them, 'Go and sit in silence, learn to understand yourself, relax mentally and reflect on the good things that you have experienced in life, and try to forget about the bad experiences.' Through meditations such as this, it is possible to feel that we are a unique part of creation, a whole, perfect and complete image of the One who has given us all life. We have to exercise a very strong conviction to become a whole being, as well as cooperating with whatever treatment we might need. Creating the right mental attitude will have a positive effect, not only on oneself, but also on the people who carry out the treatment. When we put this principle into practice, we will receive an influx of new life, which will help us to develop healing love in ourselves. This deep spiritual love should be the basis of all treatments.

Thought is a living force. Faith is creative. I often see that when patients begin to understand that I will do my best to help them in every possible way and realise the respect I have for life, and when they learn to have a little faith in me, even the weakest soon develop more trust, and harmony is established between us. Patients must not forget that in exercising the help that is given to them, they will help themselves. Love is the greatest force in the universe. That is the true sense of healing. Love is pure and has the capacity to do such tremendous things. Love and compassion are very strong forces: if we look at the tremendous amount of love that is exhibited by the greatest people on earth, we realise that this wonderful force teaches us to recognise our own sins and failures in the great light of healing, which has potency far beyond any remedy.

God is not the author of pain, disease and trouble, nor did He send this to punish His children. His great love for mankind will always be there to help. As I have often said, God will work with us; He will not work for us. We have to do our part and must exercise positive thinking. The healing powers of this will produce a harmony between mind, body and soul that will give us the power to lead a much better quality of life. The higher power will impress a will to live upon our deeper consciousness. We then find a renewal in our bodies and a more exciting life that shows the real self within us, and love beyond any understanding. We cannot learn this in one or two lessons. It will take time.

I often picture in my mind the three temples outside Peking in China: the first temple – the Temple of Supremity; the second temple – the Temple of Perfection; and the third (and most important) temple – the Temple of Harmony. The Chinese realised a long time ago that the greatest force in life is harmony between mind, body and soul, and that is what their philosophies are built on. That is basically what acupuncture does – it harmonises that which is out of harmony. How often do we see that our own thoughts disturb the harmony of the mind? The secret of health is to eliminate untrue and wrong thoughts from the mind. This is extremely important. Say to yourself, 'Health is mine, I want to be happy and healthy; I want to live my life in harmony with myself and Creation.' You will then find that happiness often follows from within.

Take some time each day to sit and meditate and visualise very strongly that you will get better. Visualise being surrounded by all that is good, and the bad forces being overpowered by pure forces. Good will always win over bad. To disconnect oneself from what is bad is the best treatment that one could ever receive. We are surrounded by a potent healing force which, although invisible, is there and we can all experience it, even when things are difficult and we sometimes pick up the wrong vibrations. The all-embracing creative spirit of love surrounds us. Let us look at nature, where everything is in harmony. Nature lets us understand our own disabilities better. In understanding our disabilities, we are on the way to victory. We become the builders of a new world, with the highest ideals, which become a new way of life. This will help the renewal of cells.

Even when things are difficult, use your intelligence to seek a more harmonious life. Then love will create a perfection that we have never experienced before. Let us realise that this earthly existence is only a training ground for something much better to come. Life can be a great deal more enjoyable when we discover these hidden powers in ourselves.

That is what Michael Gearin-Tosh writes about in *The Living Proof.* He concentrates on positive, powerful thinking to achieve better health. Certain methods helped him enormously, even the simple Chinese breathing exercises I taught him. After all, when we look at a newborn baby, we see that the baby has been given the breath of life. This will be with us for the entire time we are alive. However, we can improve our breathing through exercises. It would be helpful to visualise yourself in nature, walking around, looking at the harmony that surrounds you and thinking of the wonderful breath of life that keeps us alive, so that we can be part of this great universe. Think of the central point of the body, right under the navel. As the Chinese rightly say, 'The navel is the gateway to all that happens – it is the last part of the body that separates us from our mothers.' In that central point, the healing forces come together. If you lie down and put your left hand under the navel, on the tummy, and place the right hand on top of the left one, you will produce a magnetic force which not even the most experienced hypnotist can break through. Lying in this position, breathe through your nose deeply into the tummy, fill it with air and, without breaking the natural flow, exhale gently through the mouth. Breathe in and out, slowly into the tummy, out through the mouth. Don't break the flow of the breathing, but simply carry out this exercise rhythmically.

This exercise can be carried out in several ways. You can also do it kneeling down, putting the left hand on the tummy, under the navel, and placing the right hand on top. When in this prayer position, bow your head and breathe into the tummy and out through the mouth. Fill up the tummy like a football and breathe in and out rhythmically. Feel the way it relaxes you.

This technique is extremely useful when one gets a bit breathless, anxious, asthmatic or congested. Sitting down, stretch your feet out like railway tracks, drop your head down and let your arms and hands flop down by your side, relax and again breathe into the tummy and out through the mouth. After a short time, when a feeling of calmness envelops you, open your eyes and see the world in a different light. The healing powers of the universe are beyond understanding and great benefits can be achieved purely by exercising the breath of life that is given to us.

When you feel stressed, try this relaxation method. Tell each part of your body in turn to relax. Start with your toes, then your feet, your ankles and your knees, and gradually work your way through your whole body. Focus on each part of the body as you reach it and tell it to relax. When you have mastered this technique, you will feel totally relaxed and in true harmony with yourself and God. This is a wonderful experience for the soul. Within a short period of time, you will experience improved health. I get such wonderful reports from patients whose health has improved as a result of practising this method, which I also describe in my book *Stress and Nervous Disorders*.

These powers are available to everyone; it is just a question of intelligently using them in order to help ourselves achieve better health. Never think it is too late or that you are dying anyway – always look forward, with the thought that you are part of the great ocean of love that brought you into this world and made you a living creature.

Chapter Nine

Cancer and Complementary Therapies

Recently I was in Holland, a visit that I had kept under wraps in the hope of getting a few days' rest. This hope was short-lived, as before long a young lady appeared on my doorstep accompanied by her husband. I could see a deep sadness in the eyes of this lovely couple as they spoke about the lady's condition. It transpired that she had been through several stages of progressive lymph cancer, which had then attacked her ovaries and, ultimately, her lungs.

Deep down, she had a strong desire to survive and – rightly so – she wanted to enjoy life. Her husband was very supportive. She had been to various institutes and, in cooperation with her doctor and oncologist, had tried different therapies, but all to no avail. She undertook her regimes with the greatest efficacy and courage and yet, after each consultation, she was given the same message that there was no improvement.

I was encouraged, however, to see that she had a fairly good immune system. On the dietary front, she had undertaken several therapies but unfortunately her condition had remained unchanged. She had completed the courses of chemotherapy and radiotherapy and felt so helpless, as she was doing all she could to fight the cancer, with no results.

I wanted to treat this lady and to do my best to help her. During our talk, I uncovered a few things that, in my opinion, had been overlooked during her treatments. In the course of the several tests that I carried out, I noticed she had substantial poisonous material in her system. Although dental amalgam was not revealed to be causing a problem when we used the Vegacheck machine, on further checking, it could be seen that an aggressive chemical influence was definitely present.

I questioned her about diet. Although she had not been a smoker, test results showed that her lungs were badly affected. I also enquired in more detail about her life. It transpired that, as a young girl, she had lived in a fairly healthy part of Holland where there is low toxicity in the air. However, she did drink a lot of milk and was very fond of cheese. My mind went back to the days when I used to work in a pharmacy in that part of Holland, and how I had been extremely worried about farmers' extensive use of penicillin and certain other chemicals which were injected into cows. Disturbingly, there was very little monitoring of the amounts used, nor of the huge quantities of pesticides, insecticides and fertilisers being sprayed. While I was looking at this beautiful lady, I wondered whether some of our British doctors and professors could not argue the claim that cow's milk, which contains a lot of chemicals, also influences our hormonal system, which was certainly the case with this lady.

The fight to get chemicals banned is certainly nothing new. Although nowadays we are concerned about the health risks posed by such chemicals as Lindane, some years ago we were worried that the use of DDT had not been forbidden. As I said, being in pharmacy during that period, I was extremely concerned about the tremendous quantities of chemicals being distributed throughout the country. Sadly, that was the case not only in Holland but throughout almost the entire world. I wondered what was happening to people's health. Luckily, as time passes we are getting closer to finding answers, as diagnostic tools become more advanced. This is where complementary medicine comes into its own and can be of tremendous help to conventional medicine. For example, the Vegacheck machine, recently developed, can be used to check over the whole body and pinpoint areas that are in need of attention. In addition, this machine indicates possible reactions that may have taken place in the body.

Oncologists and doctors who have open minds regarding complementary treatments can benefit greatly from the information that can be obtained, if they are willing to listen. Although even highly qualified complementary practitioners need to leave the treatment of cancer to oncologists, they are able to help by building up the patient's strength and boosting their immune system so that the work of the conventional specialist is made easier. I have often witnessed this. Although the combination of treatments might seem to be contraindicated, they all have one thing in common – to help the cancer patients fight their battle and to get the balance right between the healthy cells and the cancer cells, by building up the healthy cells as much as possible. Those are methods that I have looked at over the years. All practitioners have a single thought – to help control cancer cells in patients in whichever way possible.

The many alternative cancer therapies available today express the personal views of every doctor and practitioner by whom they have been developed. The differences between the approaches do not take anything away from the fact that each practitioner accepts responsibility for the patients' health and will do his or her best to ease suffering and look for a method to control any problems. There are methods which have proved their worth in different situations and their application has helped cancer patients. However, one has to be very careful never to give false hope. Instead, one must look carefully at the various alternative or complementary routes to see what can be done to support whatever established conventional treatment the patient is receiving.

Dr Vogel worked very hard to develop such invaluable preparations as *Petaforce, Petasan, Viscum album* and *Echinaforce*. The principles of his treatment methods were basically improving general health. He built up the health and immune system of his patients in order to improve their health and had great success in making the patients stronger and more able to cope with some of the aggressive treatments they were receiving.

I still think that Dr Issels, the well-known German doctor who

145

treated the famous musician Jacqueline du Pré, was correct when he said:

> Cancer is not a localised disease, but a chronic, degenerative disease of the whole body. Before a tumour can grow, the body must be sick. Cells that can change to cancer exist in every person. When cancer develops, the body's defences are too weak to resist the change to the cancer cells. Tumours are a late stage in the disease. For a cure, the body's natural defence system has to be totally restored.

My friend, Dr Hans Moolenburgh, who has devoted his entire life to researching this dreadful disease, has a very sound foundation in orthodox medicine and has done a great deal to improve the general health of cancer patients. Proof of this is evident from his record of successful results. The methods that Dr Moerman practised over the years have also led to a greater understanding of cancer. When he studied cancer in pigeons, he came to three very important conclusions:

1. The high oxidation capacity of pigeons is influenced by the range of food matters that protect these birds against cancer. Therefore, specific elements in food could be an important weapon in our fight against cancer.

2. The fact that an unhealthy situation has to be present for a cancer to develop gives reason to believe that cancer could be fought with a similar method, i.e. treatment of the whole person through selected food elements.

3. Cancer arises as a result of an unsettlement in the metabolism, namely a decreased oxygenation capacity and an increase in the fermentation process, causing demolition of sugars and carbohydrates in general, without the production of oxygen, thus producing lactic acid. In other words, when cancer arises, it occurs in an internal organ with a decreased capacity for oxidation, combined with fermentation.

CANCER AND COMPLIMENTARY THERAPIES

These opinions have been applied by many others and I have met many cancer specialists throughout the world who have each, along the way, followed some of these principles: Drs Contreras, Gerson, Moerman, Manners, Moolenburgh, Kelley, Forbes and many others. As Dr Gerson once said, 'Everybody has a healing mechanism. The doctor's role is to activate it.'

The level of success achievable depends on the cooperation of the patient. In Britain, I am happy to say that since the opening of the Bristol Cancer Help Centre in July 1983, I have received tremendous cooperation, which has been reciprocated. I have had some wonderful conversations with Dr Alec Forbes, the founder of this clinic. The centre provides a complementary approach to cancer and their success is well recognised. The doctors there share my sentiments on dietary management and nutrition. I would like to mention some of their thoughts, which are very much in agreement with my own.

Their approach towards nutrition is one of healthy eating in order to strengthen the body physically, emotionally, mentally and spiritually, and to promote healthy immune and repair functions. One major consideration is that eating should be enjoyable and not in any way stressful. So, if you decide to make any changes in your diet, do so gently, exploring and enjoying the changes rather than feeling pressurised to make them. We are all unique individuals and our nutritional needs are different. The guidelines provided here are generalised and may well need to be modified according to your particular requirements.

GUIDELINES AND RECOMMENDED FOODS

Wholefood (i.e. nothing added or taken away), e.g. wholemeal bread, brown flour, brown rice
Fresh fruit and vegetables in season, lightly steamed or as salad – try to eat both daily
Raw cereals (muesli), nuts, seeds, dried fruits, etc. Try to eat some daily
Organically grown food, as available and affordable
Organic poultry, eggs, game and fish – deep-sea fish is preferable

147

to farmed fish

Beans, pulses, lentils, vegetables and cereals. These foods are also a good source of dietary fibre, but bran should be avoided as it is too irritant to the bowel

Cold-pressed oils for cooking and dressings

Variety. Avoid excessive dependence on any one food

Freshly made fruit and vegetable juices using organic fruit and vegetables

Drink lots of filtered or spring water, up to 2 litres daily if possible, not taken at the same time as meals

Avoid as much as possible: all chemically farmed fruit, vegetables, meat and eggs. In general, avoid the following:

Red meat, i.e. beef, pork, lamb, veal, bacon

Caffeine, i.e. tea, coffee, chocolate, fizzy drinks and excess alcohol

Sugar (use honey and raw sugar if necessary)

Salt

Fats and dairy produce, i.e. milk, cheese, cream and yoghurt (use soy products instead)

Smoked or pickled foods

Preservatives and additives

Mouldy or damaged food

Food which has been stored for long periods, irradiated, dried, processed, microwaved or repeatedly reheated

Margarines and fats/spreads containing hydrogenated fats (among those not containing hydrogenated fats is Vitaquel)

How you feel about your food and whether you are enjoying it are very important – so there is no need to let your diet become a penance! Give yourself time to eat slowly, enjoy your meals and relax afterwards if possible. If you have particular problems with eating, you should consult a holistic doctor or nutritional therapist.

I also admire Pat Pilkington, co-founder of the Bristol Cancer Help Centre, whose dedication through her hard work has been a great comfort and help to so many people attending the clinic. Combining a nutritional approach with specific remedies has been extremely beneficial in helping those suffering from this monstrous disease.

Responsible practitioners and researchers are at work all over the world, but their goal is the same – how best to help people who suffer. We all recognise the need for a sensible diet, eliminating waste products from the system, fighting degenerative cells and helping people towards better health. The responsibility is ours – patients and practitioners alike. We have to combine body, mind and spirit to fight cancer.

Basically, it doesn't cost much to change one's diet and, as extra protection, add some homoeopathic, herbal, or vitamin and mineral therapies to your regime. It is very important that the patient follows the practitioner's advice – as did a 28-year-old female who consulted me. She was suffering from ovarian cancer, had very low energy and had also developed kidney problems. It is often said that the kidneys are the seat of the emotions and when I looked closer into this young woman's life, I could see that she had endured a series of mishaps since the birth of her last child. She was on several drugs at that time. She was having a lot of problems with her husband and emotional trauma with his parents and, as a consequence, her kidneys had started to play up and energy blockages were very noticeable. She was pushing herself to get on top of this, when suddenly she went downhill very quickly. This resulted in metabolic problems, swelling in her legs, diarrhoea and depression, and she needed urgent help. I prescribed a few strong homoeopathic remedies to stop her constant diarrhoea, the kidney pain and to enable her to get some sleep. The next time I saw her, I noticed that the swelling in her legs had gone down, she was sleeping more soundly and her metabolic system had started to improve. I then prescribed some strong antioxidants to boost her energy, together with some acupuncture treatment. After that, I cooperated with what her oncologist was doing and started to treat her with *Petasites* and *IP-6* with *inositol*, after which she started to feel better. Her liver also needed treatment. At the risk of repeating myself, I must emphasise once more that wherever the cancer is located, the liver is always involved and needs treatment. An all-round general improvement soon became noticeable with this young woman and her home situation also improved. She became calmer, much more patient and gained control over her domestic problems. Luckily, her depression lifted, her circulation improved, her condition became more controllable and today she feels much better.

There are many ways in which you can approach such situations by the introduction of complementary methods. Every doctor, consultant or practitioner will be grateful for an intelligent input to boost the cancer patient's health. It is really worthwhile to make every effort, to make sure that one is doing everything possible – not only to ease the problem, but also to strive to give the cancer patient a better quality of life.

Conclusion

As I was nearing the end of writing this book, I received a phone call from a woman who I greatly admire and regard as being one of the most intelligent people in public life. She has appeared on radio and television, and possesses many fine qualities. Having known her since she was a child, she has matured into a most attractive lady. She is a young mother, happily married and has a good relationship with her family.

However, something happened in her life that greatly disturbed her and a short time later, she consulted me for advice on a small lump she had discovered in her breast. As this caused me concern, I advised her to have it investigated. Unfortunately, the lump was indeed malignant. Immediate action was taken by the hospital, with the addition of some therapies and remedies I prescribed. She was very positive and focused on one thing – this would not beat her. I gave her advice on several aspects and even arranged for her to see my friend Dr Hans Moolenburgh in Holland, who also examined her thoroughly. Sadly, some of her lymph glands were affected and every possible action needed to be taken. I admired her for the terrific input she gave, by following a restricted diet and taking the remedies we mutually agreed. Indeed, she coped extremely well. Like so many others, she got a terrific shock when she discovered she had cancer. However, she took the problem in hand with a positive attitude and said to me, 'I shall not be beaten by this horrible disease. I shall fight it to the end.' That is precisely what she has been doing. Although she has had several setbacks and has been battling courageously to overcome cancer, the contented inward spirit she possesses proves extremely helpful during times of tremendous difficulty.

I would reiterate that a cancer cell is like a brain cell. She influenced these cells with her positive spirit and tackled her cancer on the principles that I have written about in previous chapters. The more physical attacks she coped with, the more she grew spiritually. With the help of her husband, her parents and many friends, she battles very bravely and has, thankfully, a good quality of life. This is probably one of the most aggressive cancers I have encountered but, by remaining spiritually strong, she effectively keeps the condition under control, emotionally and mentally. She is, as she herself says, a much stronger person in herself than she was before.

Spiritual growth can offer great encouragement to those who are suffering. Cancer patients who possess a fighting spirit often overcome physical traumas. Conversely, those who are negative and believe that because they have cancer nothing can be done and they are going to die anyway, are spiritually weak. They have an extremely short-sighted outlook and can become so miserable that they do eventually die. What is important is to pick up the pieces and gather the strength to deal with the problem head-on.

'Cure' is a very big word. Degenerative diseases such as diabetes, arthritis and cancer can be controlled to a great extent, to enable people to lead fairly normal lives. This is entirely different to those diseases that can actually be cured. It is not a good idea to mislead patients and give them false hope. It is more beneficial for the patient to be realistic and say, 'I will do everything in my power to control the cancer, and trust those people that are of similar minds.'

Another young woman who came to see me had been prescribed HRT in order to control a hormonal imbalance. Unfortunately, the HRT had the opposite effect and resulted in her developing breast cancer. She came to see me and was very bitter about this. I tried to put her mind at rest by saying it was probably

CONCLUSION

not the HRT that had caused the cancer, but that it had triggered off something already within her body. I told her that it would be pointless to remain angry, as anger is one of the worst things for provoking cancer but, instead, she should accept that this had happened and make the best of it by tackling this disease with my help. I usually say this to patients who dwell on trying to work out what could have caused them to develop cancer. It is extremely difficult to find an answer. It would be wonderful if we could simply compare it to an Agatha Christie novel, where the answer is found on the last page. Unfortunately, there are still many question marks over the whole subject.

Scientific surveys have proved an association between pain and cancer, but we can never say that pain is a precancerous condition. The signs and symptoms might be clear enough, but the establishment of cancer is something different. Much investigation is still needed into how long this process takes. It is notable that over $20 billion has been spent on cancer research in the United States, with state-of-the-art equipment being used in an attempt to ascertain the possible causes of cancer.

Numerous questions still need answers: for instance, can cancer be reversed? What are the clinically proven complementary and alternative therapies? Most importantly, can orthodox medicine and alternative medicine be combined to alleviate the terrible suffering surrounding this monstrous disease? There is no doubt that worldwide concern on the whole subject has become more intense and there is now greater acceptance of the statement that cancer is a metabolic disease which can be greatly influenced by dietary management.

When strengthening the immune system, herbs, homoeopathic remedies and vitamins, minerals and trace elements play an enormously important. It is fascinating to read the story of Essiac and Hoxsey, who were both deeply involved in cancer research, and discovered by chance that some cancers disappeared when they used specific herbs. These herbs are extremely useful in cancer cases, whether in humans or animals.

The importance of research groups throughout the world is paramount. Study groups and research have to be promoted, with money being made available for this invaluable work. We saw this in a recent study of workers following an explosion at a nuclear power station in Russia. When the herb *Gingko biloba* was administered over a two-month period, a decrease of two-thirds in the chromosome damage was reported. Such damage can lead to cancer so the conclusions were interesting. In another study on malignant melanomas, during a series of six ninety-minute support group meetings, it was reported that the cancer patients became less depressed and a significantly lower rate of recurrence was noted. It is therefore essential that support groups throughout the world obtain all the necessary funding.

Groups who have carried out studies on the prevention of cancer have all come to one conclusion – detoxification is necessary. We see how beneficial this is even with very simple liver flushes, coffee enemas, colon cleansing and the correct dietary combination of essential fatty acids. It is very much up to all practitioners or institutes who treat cancer patients in a complementary way to ensure that multi-disciplinary programmes are devised for each individual patient. Every symptom should be looked at logically. Every cancer patient should be treated as an individual in a holistic system.

I greatly admire the work of Dr W. John Diamond. He said, 'I do not treat cancer so much as I treat patients who have cancer as a prime physical manifestation. This is the essential distinction between an orthodox and alternative approach to cancer treatment. An orthodox approach seeks to destroy the tumour while the approach of the alternative physician seeks to treat the patient and enable the patient's system to destroy the tumour.' I concur with Dr Diamond's belief that cancer should be treated holistically: it is important to treat not only the physical, but also the mental and the emotional states, as well as the cancerous tumour, in whatever treatment is chosen.

When cancer patients attend regular check-ups, I am often encouraged by the terrific change in the readings of their tests when they are being prescribed certain complementary remedies. Early treatment is necessary when cancer is detected and the quicker treatment is undertaken the better. The success of combining complementary medicine and conventional oncology has been proven many times. An efficacious approach in reversing cancer and preventing future recurrence is important. It is said that no single therapy, method or substance can treat cancer due to the complexity of the disease.

I have found over the years that cancer patients are usually most cooperative. They are aware of the complex nature of the problem and the vast majority are eager to do all they can to help in their fight. This positive approach is of great benefit in the treatment of the disease. It is amazing how one particular treatment can sometimes turn the situation around and have a positive result on their condition.

I always respected Dr Contreras who worked with us in our clinic in Troon in Scotland for a short time. He demonstrated how conditions could change enormously with the small amount of remedies he used, and how effectively his application aided even terminally ill cancer patients. With great admiration, I watched him work holistically on the patient in a similar way to Dr Vogel and Dr Moerman. That devotion encourages me to fight on and continue to help patients who are suffering.

The young lady I spoke of at the beginning of this conclusion said a wise thing when we were talking late one evening: once she was diagnosed with cancer, she took a good look at herself and began to learn more about her character. She then began to look at her life with a more positive attitude, to ensure that she overcame the gradual degeneration in her body by influencing it with the introduction of the many methods she applied. I admire her for the way in which she faced her problems, for whenever she thought of a positive way in which to adapt some part of her programme, she took appropriate action. That is the reason she is still alive today and maintains a quality of life that she would otherwise have lost long ago.

We live in a polluted world, with viruses, parasites, bacteria, allergies, deficiencies . . . one could go on and on. It is crucial that we adopt a positive attitude towards difficult situations. However, this can only be done if we take care of our bodies, physically, mentally and emotionally. A strong immune system can stop cancer cells in their tracks.

FEMALE CANCERS

There are many books on the subject of cancer and many methods of treatment. As I have said, it is difficult to decide which method to choose. It is important when taking the alternative approach to look for a practitioner with many years' experience in the field, as I have often seen patients in a state of panic after having taken every remedy possible and almost killing themselves with what they thought would help. Using remedies that were incompatible probably exacerbated their problems, as they did not possess the necessary ingredients. However, I was always encouraged at the annual meetings of the Cancer Control Society in Los Angeles when survivors came up and gave their testimonies on how they had survived, which methods they followed and how they adapted different methods for their own individual needs. Usually with great enthusiasm, they related stories of how they had made either physical or emotional adjustments to their lives, and how this healing process had improved their quality of life.

This book gives a glimpse of some of the treatments I have used over the years. During this time, the advice I have imparted has given innumerable patients relief from their suffering, a better quality of life and, in some cases, has even helped them overcome disastrous conditions. Every single person on earth today is exposed to innumerable toxic chemicals and pollutions in the three forms of energy by which we live – food, water and air. Toxicity is greatly on the increase and every time I study patients' blood tests or use the Vegacheck machine I am amazed at how much waste material is present in the human body. These bodies of ours, which are fields of energy, have to be examined to determine where the energies have been disturbed, what is influencing these energies and what could be the cause. I repeat that prevention is better than cure. To everyone who is affected by cancer, be positive, fight it and do everything possible to overcome obstacles on the road to recovery.

Index

INDEX